CA

Obstetrics

IN *focus*

CW00919307

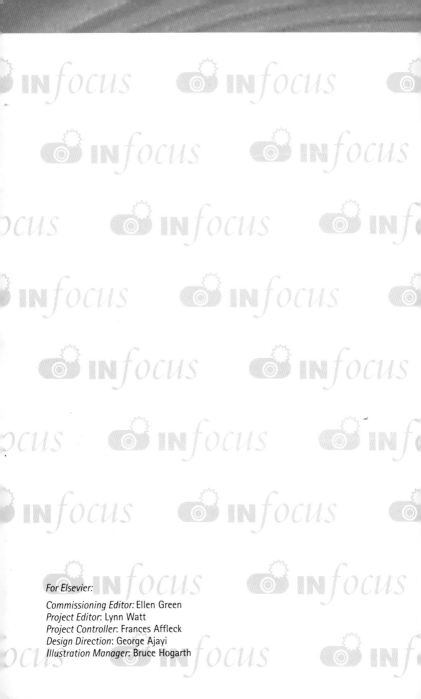

For Elsevier:

Commissioning Editor: Ellen Green
Project Editor: Lynn Watt
Project Controller: Frances Affleck
Design Direction: George Ajayi
Illustration Manager: Bruce Hogarth

Obstetrics

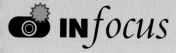 IN *focus*

David K James MA MD FRCOG DCH

Professor of Fetomaternal Medicine and Director of Medical Education
School of Human Development
Faculty of Medicine and Health Sciences
University of Nottingham
Queen's Medical Centre
Nottingham, UK

Alec McEwan MRCOG

Subspecialty Trainee in Fetal and Maternal Medicine
Queen's Medical Centre
University Hospital NHS Trust
Nottingham, UK

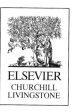

ELSEVIER
CHURCHILL
LIVINGSTONE

EDINBURGH   LONDON   NEW YORK   OXFORD   PHILADELPHIA   ST LOUIS   SYDNEY   TORONTO 2005

ELSEVIER | CHURCHILL LIVINGSTONE

An imprint of Elsevier Limited

First published 2005

ISBN 0443 074356

British Library Cataloguing in Publication Data
A catalogue record for this book is available from the British Library

Library of Congress Cataloging in Publication Data
A catalog record for this book is available from the Library of Congress

Notice
Medical knowledge is constantly changing. Standard safety precautions must be followed, but as new research and clinical experience broaden our knowledge, changes in treatment and drug therapy may become necessary or appropriate. Readers are advised to check the most current product information provided by the manufacturer of each drug to be administered to verify the recommended dose, the method and duration of administration, and contraindications. It is the responsibility of the practitioner, relying on experience and knowledge of the patient, to determine dosages and the best treatment for each individual patient. Neither the Publisher nor the authors assume any liability for any injury and/or damage to persons or property arising from this publication.

The Publisher

 ELSEVIER your source for books, journals and multimedia in the health sciences

www.elsevierhealth.com

The publisher's policy is to use paper manufactured from sustainable forests

Printed in China

Preface

We hope this illustrated book of Obstetrics, written in a concise format and supplemented with questions and answers, will appeal to medical students, nurses and midwives during the obstetrics part of their training. Pictures that illustrate important aspects of conditions are always an important supplement to clinical experience, since the range of conditions that students see is necessarily limited and subject to chance. We have therefore focused on conditions that can be clearly shown in photographs and scans, and we hope that the pictures, as well as the questions and answers, will be helpful and stimulating to students.

David James
Alec McEwan

Acknowledgements

We are grateful to the following for providing some of the illustrations for this book: Professor G.M. Stirrat, Dr B. Spiedal, Mr P. Savage, Dr P. Burton, Dr R. Slade, Dr D. Warnock, Dr A. Jeffcote, Dr N. Hunter, Dr C. Harman, Dr J. Haworth, Dr H. Andrews, Miss D. Freer, Dr S. Rosevear, Dr C. Kennedy, Dr J. Zuccollo, Dr J. Pardey, Professor W. Irving, Dr T. Jaspan, Dr J. Padfield, Mrs E. Bradley, Professor G. Enders, Dr M. R. Howard and Dr P. J. Hamilton. We are especially indebted to Mr N. Bowyer of the Department of Medical illustration, Southmead Hospital, Bristol, and Mr N. Bullimore, Department of Obstetrics, Queen's Medical Centre, Nottingham for advice and practical help in the preparation of illustrations.

2004
DJ AM

Contents

Contents

Fertilization and implantation

Fertilization of the ovum by sperm occurs in the outer third of the fallopian tube. The division of the conceptus reaches a four-cell stage after 36-48 h (Fig 1). The blastocyst arrives in the uterus at 72-96 h (16 cells) and remains free in the uterine cavity for 4-5 days.

Implantation occurs 6-9 days after fertilization. Primitive chorionic villi develop at 13-15 days. The gestation sac is visible on vaginal ultrasound 4-5 weeks after the first day of the last menstrual period (i.e. 2-3 weeks postconception) (Fig 2), and a yolk sac soon after this.

Early diagnosis of pregnancy

Human chorionic gonadotrophin (hCG) is a glycoprotein hormone secreted by the trophoblastic cells of the placenta. It is present in the urine and serum of pregnant women and is the definitive test for diagnosing pregnancy.

Assays using monoclonal antibodies are quick, simple and sensitive and can now reliably detect as little as 25-50 mU/mL of hCG—the level found approximately 10-14 days after conception.

The expected date of delivery (EDD) is 280 days after the first day of the last menstrual period (LMP) (Naegele's rule). There is some ethnic variation in the length of normal pregnancy but only by a few days.

This method of calculating the EDD from the LMP assumes conception was 2 weeks after the LMP. Conception is likely to occur later with a long cycle (e.g. 35, 42 days), irregular periods, or recent oral contraceptive use. Also, memory of the date of the LMP is often poor. Because fetal size shows little variability in the first 16 weeks of pregnancy, ultrasound may help clarify the EDD in such cases by measuring either the crown–rump length (Fig 3) or biparietal diameter.

Later, genetic and environmental factors such as maternal diabetes, infections, drug use and pre-eclampsia cause significant variation in fetal size at any particular gestation, making 'late' dating by ultrasound imprecise.

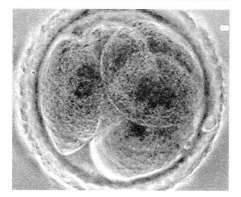

Fig 1 Blastocyst: four-cell stage.

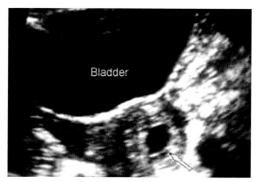

Fig 2 Ultrasound of intrauterine gestation sac (5 weeks) (arrowed).

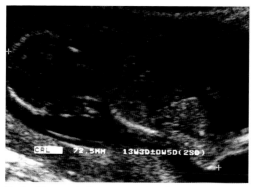

Fig 3 Ultrasound of crown–rump length.

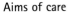

2 Normal pregnancy and care

Normal pregnancy and care

Aims of care

Pregnancy in most cases will be a normal event with low risk of harm to mother or baby. For a few, however, there is a greater risk of adverse outcomes. The aims of antenatal care are:

- To provide advice, reassurance, education and support for the woman and her family.
- To deal with minor ailments of pregnancy.
- To provide general health screening.
- To prevent, detect and manage those factors that adversely affect the health of mother and/or baby.

By repeated history-taking, examination and investigations the level of risk in a pregnancy is regularly reviewed and modifications to 'routine' care are made in the light of this.

Visits

Recent evidence-based guidelines from the National Institute of Clinical Excellence (NICE) have recommended a reduction in the number of antenatal appointments in low-risk pregnancies (first visit at 8-14 weeks, followed by visits at 20, 24, 28, 30, 32, 34, 36, 38, 40 and 41 weeks). Care is provided either solely by the general practitioner and community midwife or in combination with a consultant obstetrician ('shared care').

History

At the first ('booking') visit, the following data are recorded: maternal age, marital status, ethnic background, menstrual, medical, psychiatric, surgical, obstetric, family and social histories and details of any other problems. Drug intake, alcohol and smoking habits are also documented. The use of structured maternity records (usually carried by pregnant women) reduces the chances that identifiable risk factors will be missed. At subsequent visits any new problems are noted, together with maternal perception of fetal movements.

   Physiological changes occurring in pregnancy may cause a multitude of symptoms. Most organ systems may be involved: gastrointestinal (nausea, vomiting, oesophagitis, constipation, haemorrhoids, gum hypertrophy) (Fig 4); urogenital (urinary frequency); breasts (tingling, enlargement, nipple pigmentation) (Fig 5); skin (increased pigmentation) (Fig 6); cardiorespiratory (palpitations,

4

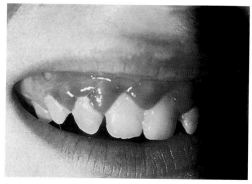

Fig 4 Gum hypertrophy.

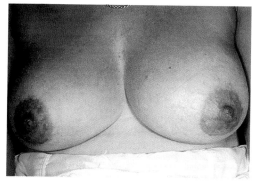

Fig 5 Breast changes.

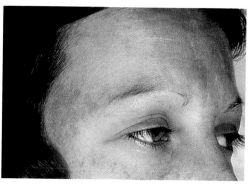

Fig 6 Chloasma (facial pigmentation).

breathlessness); and neurological (carpal tunnel syndrome). Other symptoms may indicate pathology (e.g. headaches and abdominal pain; distinguishing the two may be difficult).

Examination
At the booking visit, calculation of the body mass index and measurement of the blood pressure (BP) are important. Cardiorespiratory, breast and pelvic examinations are only necessary in those with risk factors or symptoms. At all visits, BP and uterine size are recorded. In later pregnancy, the fetal lie and presentation and the engagement of the fetal head are noted and the fetal heart is auscultated.

Signs
Early signs of pregnancy include changes in the breasts (enlargement, pigmentation, venous engorgement and Montgomery's tubercles) (Fig 5) and genitalia (bluish coloration of vaginal skin and cervix, softening and enlargement of uterus). Other signs include gum hypertrophy (Fig 4), chloasma (Fig 6), striae gravidarum (Fig 7), linea nigra, umbilical pigmentation and eversion (Fig 8), lymphadenopathy, thyroid enlargement and varicose veins (Fig 9).

Investigations
At the first visit, urinalysis is undertaken (testing for glucose, protein, ketones) and a midstream sample of urine is sent for culture. Blood is taken for complete blood count and film, ABO and rhesus typing, antibody screening, rubella antibody status and serological tests for syphilis, hepatitis B and HIV. Haemoglobin electrophoresis is indicated if the woman is Afro-American/Caribbean, Mediterranean, or from the Far East. At 16 weeks, biochemical screening tests may be performed for fetal neural tube defects and Down syndrome. Some units offer screening for Down syndrome by fetal nuchal translucency measurement at 11-13 weeks (Fig 29). Urinalysis is performed at all subsequent visits, and haemoglobin and red cell antibody screening is repeated at 28 and 34 weeks.

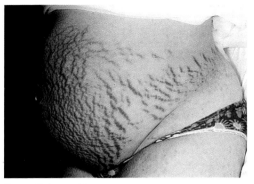

Fig 7   Striae gravidarum.

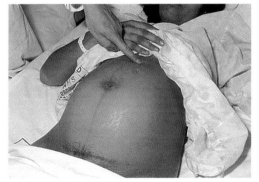

Fig 8   Linea nigra and umbilical pigmentation and eversion.

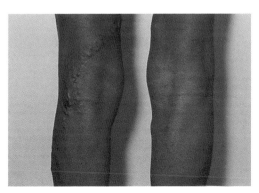

Fig 9   Varicose veins.

Miscarriage

Definition
Expulsion of the products of conception before the 24th week of pregnancy (20th week in USA) in which the fetus shows no signs of life after delivery. Most miscarriages occur in the first 12 weeks. Miscarriage occurs in 15-20% of clinically detected pregnancies. Recurrent miscarriage is defined as three or more consecutive spontaneous miscarriages.

Classification
- *Threatened*: vaginal bleeding but pregnancy continues.
- *Inevitable*: vaginal bleeding, uterine contractions (pain) and an open cervical os, but before the passage of products of conception.
- *Incomplete*: pregnancy tissues have been passed per vaginum, but the uterus is not yet empty. The cervical os is open (Fig 10).
- *Complete*: all the products of conception have been expelled, the uterus is empty and the cervix is closed.
- *Missed*: an ultrasound diagnosis. No heart beat is visible in a fetus with a crown–rump length of ≥6 mm (Fig 11).
- *Anembryonic pregnancy (blighted ovum)*: an empty gestation sac measuring ≥20 mm on ultrasound.

Aetiology
Often no cause is apparent. However, if investigated, fetal abnormalities (especially chromosomal) are the most common cause. Others include phospholipid syndromes (e.g. lupus), thrombophilias, polycystic ovary syndrome, congenital uterine anomalies, cytotoxic drugs, cervical incompetence (second trimester losses).

Clinical features
Amenorrhea, colicky pain (40%), bleeding (variable in amount) (98%), shock (5%), cervical dilation and passage of products (15%), chance ultrasound finding.

Management
Making a diagnosis may be difficult at early gestations and repeated scanning is often necessary. Management can be conservative, medical (using antiprogestogens) or surgical (Fig 12). The choice is determined by the clinical features and patient's wishes.

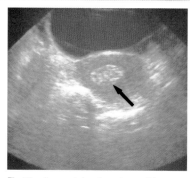

Fig 10 Incomplete miscarriage with retained products of conception.

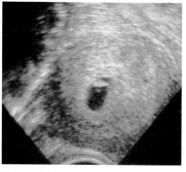

Fig 11 Vaginal ultrasound of missed miscarriage.

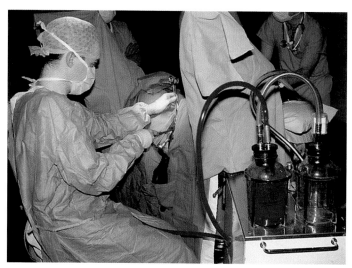

Fig 12 Surgical evacuation of retained products of conception.

Ectopic pregnancy

Definition
Implantation of a pregnancy in a site other than the normal uterine cavity (Fig 13). Occurs in 1% of pregnancies. The most common site is the ampullary portion of the fallopian tube (Fig 14). Other sites include the ovary and abdomen.

Aetiology
Risk factors include tubal damage (secondary to pelvic infection, tubal reconstructive surgery and a previous ectopic pregnancy), use of intrauterine contraceptive devices and assisted reproductive techniques.

Clinical features
Symptoms   Lower abdominal pain (usually unilateral), bleeding (often dark red vaginal 'spotting'), dizziness and shoulder tip pain (subdiaphragmatic irritation by intraperitoneal blood).

Signs   Hypotension and tachycardia out of proportion to the visible bleeding, cervical excitation, adnexal tenderness and sometimes a mass. Tubal rupture will produce sudden pain followed by shock and collapse.

Investigations
A combination of transvaginal ultrasound scanning and measurement of serum human chorionic gonadotrophin (hCG) levels avoids excessive use of laparoscopy for making the diagnosis. An intrauterine gestation sac should be visible with hCG levels greater than 1500 IU/L. The majority of intrauterine ongoing pregnancies will demonstrate a greater than 66% rise in hCG levels over 48 h. Most ectopic pregnancies do not.

Management
Depends on clinical features, vaginal ultrasound findings and serum hCG levels. Options include:
- *Medical.* Intramuscular methotrexate is reserved for compliant women with minimal symptoms, no cardiovascular compromise and small ectopics.
- *Surgical.* The most common treatment is laparoscopic or open salpingotomy (conservative surgery) or salpingectomy (removal of the affected tube) (Fig 15). Salpingectomy is currently favoured if the other tube appears normal because salpingotomy carries a risk of persistent trophoblast and higher future ectopic rate.

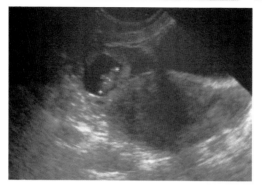

Fig 13   Vaginal ultrasound showing ectopic pregnancy with the fetus above and to the left of the empty uterus.

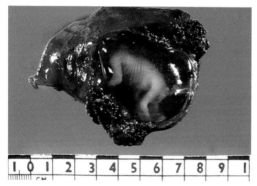

Fig 14   Pathology specimen of ectopic pregnancy.

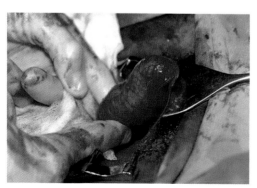

Fig 15   Tubal ectopic pregnancy at laparotomy.

Trophoblastic disease

Definition
Neoplasia occurring in the placenta.

Incidence
1 in 600 pregnancies in the Far East, but 1 in 2000 in the West.

Pathology
The villi become grossly hydropic. The majority are benign (hydatidiform mole) but have pseudomalignant properties, capable of myometrial invasion and systemic dissemination. In a 'complete' mole (Fig 16) no fetus is present. The karyotype is diploid (46 chromosomes) but the chromosomes are totally paternal in origin. Rarely, a complete mole can become malignant (choriocarcinoma). A 'partial' mole (Fig 17) is always found in association with a triploid fetus (69 chromosomes) with the extra set of chromosomes being of paternal origin. Partial moles do not normally become malignant.

Clinical features
Uterine bleeding, exaggerated features of pregnancy, a larger than expected uterus and the passage of grape-like tissue per vaginum. Pre-eclampsia and thyrotoxicosis may complicate the clinical picture.

Diagnosis
Often made at curettage for presumed incomplete miscarriage. A characteristic placental 'snowstorm' appearance on ultrasound (Fig 18) and very high hCG levels often point to the diagnosis beforehand.

Investigations
Tissue for histology and karyotype; chest radiograph; serum hCG; thyroid, liver and renal function; complete blood count; ABO and rhesus group.

Management
The uterus is emptied by suction and curettage. Subsequent monitoring of urinary and/or serum hCG levels is supervised by one of the three national trophoblast centres. Levels that fail to fall or subsequently rise again suggest incomplete evacuation, invasion, metastasis or malignant change. Chemotherapy with methotrexate is usually curative and hysterectomy is rarely indicated. Avoidance of pregnancy for at least a year is strongly advised.

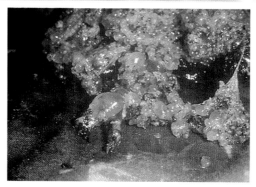

Fig 16   Complete mole.

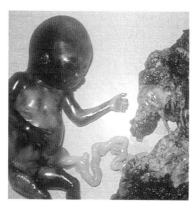

Fig 17   Partial mole with triploid fetus.

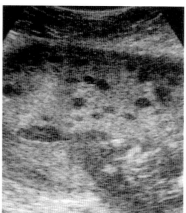

Fig 18   Ultrasound picture of a partial mole (multiple echolucent areas in the placenta but with fetal parts also).

Rubella

Mother
Incubation period of 2-3 weeks. Maculopapular rash
(Fig 19), lymphadenopathy, fever, malaise, conjunctivitis and
cough. Diagnosed by finding rubella-specific IgM antibody
(falls after 3 months) or rising titres of IgG. Virus can be
cultured from a throat swab.

Non-immune women should be offered postnatal
vaccination. Inadvertent vaccination in early pregnancy has
not been associated with congenital disease.

Baby
First trimester fetal infection carries an 80-90% risk of
damage in survivors, including eye (Fig 20) and cardiac
defects, microcephaly, mental retardation, thrombocytopenic
purpura, hepatosplenomegaly and growth restriction. Second
trimester infection causes sensorineural deafness in 10-15%.

Toxoplasmosis

Mother
Often asymptomatic. Risk factors include contact with cats
and ingestion of undercooked meat. Diagnosed by finding
toxoplasma-specific IgM on serological testing.

Baby
Fetal infection occurs in a minority of cases (20%) with
15% developing congenital abnormalities, including growth
restriction, chorioretinitis, hydrocephalus and intracranial
calcification. Thrombocytopenic purpura,
hepatosplenomegaly, jaundice, fever, pneumonitis and
convulsions may be apparent at birth.

Granulomatous lesions (Fig 21), pseudocysts and
calcification occur in the central nervous system, eyes,
lungs, heart, liver, spleen and kidneys.

Syphilis

Mother
The risk of fetal infection varies with stage of maternal
disease: 90% with primary (chancre) and secondary
(disseminated lymphadenopathy and rash) infection; 40%
with latent infection; and 10% with late (gummas,

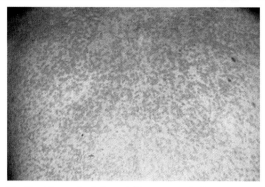

Fig 19   Maternal rubella rash (German measles).

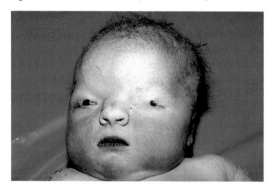

Fig 20   Rubella-induced microphthalmia.

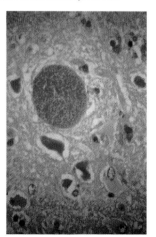

Fig 21   Toxoplasma body within the fetal brain.

neurological and cardiovascular) infection. Diagnosis is by isolation of the organism (primary and secondary) and serological tests. Seropositive mothers are usually treated with penicillin.

Baby

A quarter of fetal syphilis infections end in fetal loss, a quarter in preterm labour or fetal growth restriction and half in a congenitally infected neonate. Associated ultrasound findings may include hydrops, polyhydramnios or hepatomegaly. Amniotic fluid or fetal blood can be tested directly for *Treponema pallidum*. Most newborns are asymptomatic; however a few will manifest early congenital syphilis (rash, hepatosplenomegaly, lymphadenopathy, oedema). Treatment is with penicillin.

Cytomegalovirus

Mother

Almost always asymptomatic. If cytomegalovirus (CMV) is suspected, then isolation of the virus from cervix or urine is possible. CMV can reactivate, posing minimal risk to the fetus.

Baby

The fetus becomes infected in 30-40% of primary maternal infections. Of those infected, 5-7% will be symptomatic at birth, with thrombocytopenic purpura (Fig 22), hepatosplenomegaly, chorioretinitis, microphthalmia, nephritis, microcephaly, deafness, mental retardation, cerebral calcifications and growth restriction. Diagnosis is by isolation of the virus.

Histologically, CMV-infected cells frequently have cytoplasmic inclusions (virus particles surrounded by lysosomes) (Fig 23).

Parvovirus

Mother

Fever, malaise and rarely postinfectious arthralgia. 20% of adult infections are asymptomatic.

Baby

Fetal infection can cause an aplastic crisis, with anaemia, myocarditis and hydrops fetalis (Fig 24). In the second trimester, fetal loss rates may reach 1 in 10, occurring 4-6 weeks after exposure. The risk after 20 weeks is significantly less. Fetal anaemia can be treated with intrauterine transfusions.

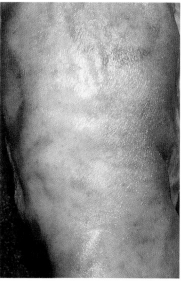

Fig 22 Cytomegalovirus (CMV): cutaneous manifestations in the trunk.

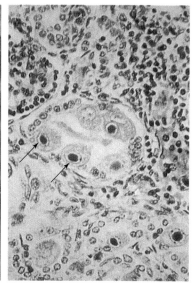

Fig 23 Cytomegalovirus (CMV): inclusion bodies found within the fetal kidney.

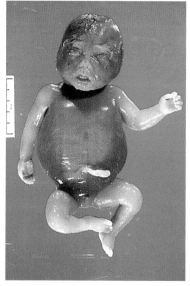

Fig 24 Fetal parvovirus infection causing hydrops.

Varicella zoster (chickenpox)

Mother

Symptoms include fever, malaise and a pruritic maculopapular rash which becomes widespread and vesicular. Incubation period is 10-20 days and transmission is through respiratory droplets. Individuals are infectious 48 h before the rash appears. A pneumonitis occurs in 10% of adults and is said to be fatal in as many as 6%. Maternal infection may be prevented by administration of varicella immunoglobulin (VZIG) and the disease itself ameliorated by the use of aciclovir.

Baby

The congenital varicella syndrome occurs in 1-2% of pregnancies when maternal infection occurs at less than 20 weeks' gestation. It comprises microcephaly, cortical atrophy, limb hypoplasia (Fig 25) and severe skin scarring; VZIG probably reduces this risk. Peripartum infection may result in a serious neonatal varicella infection (widespread skin rash (Fig 26), thrombocytopenia, hepatosplenomegaly, jaundice, meningoencephalitis). Asymptomatic newborns may later present with 'shingles', representing a reactivation of their in utero infection (Fig 27).

Listeriosis

Mother

Infection with *Listeria monocytogenes* is usually asymptomatic, occasionally producing a flu-like illness with abdominal pain and diarrhoea. Eating unpasteurized dairy products and raw vegetables should be avoided. Treatment is with ampicillin.

Baby

Congenital infection only occurs with very heavy colonization. Miscarriage may occur in early pregnancy, stillbirth later on. Survivors develop either an early- or late-onset disease pattern. In the former, diffuse septicaemia causes cutaneous (Fig 28), pulmonary, hepatic and neurological lesions (mortality 90%). Late-onset infection, possibly acquired after birth, is characterized by meningitis, with mental retardation and/or hydrocephalus (mortality 40%).

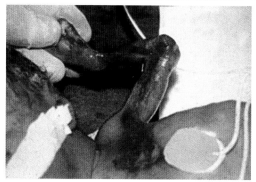

Fig 25   Limb hypoplasia secondary to fetal varicella infection. Reproduced with permission from Gisela Enders, Institute for Virology, Infectiology and Epidemiology, Stuttgart.

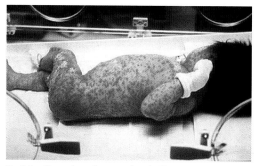

Fig 26   Disseminated neonatal varicella.

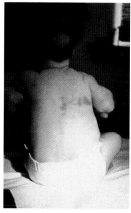

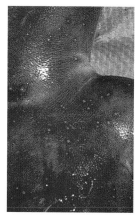

Fig 27   Herpes zoster ('shingles').   Fig 28   Listeriosis: cutaneous manifestations.

Prenatal diagnosis

General

Over the past 20 years, dramatic advances have been made in prenatal diagnosis.

Fetal imaging

The resolution of ultrasound (Fig 29) has improved significantly and MRI can be used for difficult cases (see Ch 7).

Obstetric procedures

These are performed under ultrasound control and include chorionic villus sampling (placental biopsy), amniocentesis, fetal blood sampling and fetal tissue biopsy.

Laboratory methods

These include chromosome analysis (karyotyping) of metaphase cells either directly or after fetal cell culture, DNA analysis, enzyme assay and measurement of haematological values. Fluorescence in situ hybridization (FISH) (Fig 30) is a relatively new molecular technique used for counting chromosomes in interphase cells; major aneuploidies can be excluded or confirmed within 24-48 h.

Chorionic villus sampling

Procedures

Biopsy or aspiration of cells can be achieved using transabdominal (Fig 31) or transcervical routes, the former being more commonly practised.

Chorionic villi (Fig 32) may be used for chromosome analysis, DNA analysis (e.g. cystic fibrosis, haemoglobinopathies, Duchenne muscular dystrophy) and enzymology (inborn errors of metabolism).

Risks

The risk is dependent on gestational age. The earlier in pregnancy, the higher the risk of miscarriage (e.g. about 2% at 11 weeks and about 1% at 16 weeks). Additional risks include membrane rupture, infection, rhesus sensitization and uterine trauma. Chorionic villus sampling is rarely performed before 10 weeks because of the risk of limb defects.

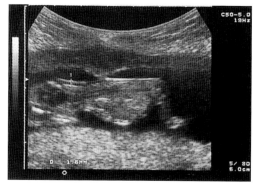

Fig 29   Nuchal translucency.

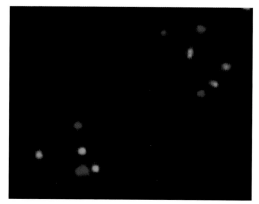

Fig 30   FISH study showing two triploid cells (three copies of each chromosome).

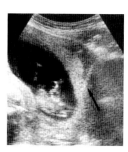

Fig 31   Transabdominal chorionic villus sampling (needle arrowed).

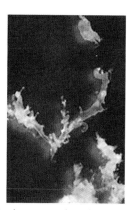

Fig 32   Low-power view of chorionic villi.

Amniocentesis

Procedure
Amniotic fluid is obtained by inserting an 18-20-gauge spinal needle into the amniotic cavity transabdominally under ultrasound guidance (Figs 33-35). It is performed after the first trimester, usually at 16 weeks.

Indications
Chromosome analysis (for chromosomal abnormalities, fetal sexing in X-linked conditions), inborn errors of metabolism (enzymes, metabolites using cells or supernatant), DNA analysis (if there is a gene probe for a specific condition) and later in pregnancy for assessment of rhesus disease (see Ch 9).

Risks
Amniocentesis after 15 weeks carries a miscarriage risk of 1.0%. If performed at earlier gestations there is a greater risk of respiratory distress and postural deformities. Amniocentesis at later gestations may cause preterm rupture of membranes, chorioamnionitis and preterm labour. Rhesus sensitization can occur at any time (as with any of these invasive techniques) and rhesus-negative women must have a Kleihauer test performed and anti-D immunoglobulin given.

Fetal blood sampling and other techniques

Fetal blood can be aspirated from the umbilical cord after 18 weeks' gestation, although alternative sites are sometimes chosen (e.g. intrahepatic part of the umbilical vein) (Fig 36). Fetal blood may be required to diagnose/investigate inherited haemoglobin disorders, inborn errors of metabolism, chromosomal anomalies, fetal viral infections, rhesus disease, unexplained hydrops and fetal anaemia. Risks include miscarriage, trauma, blood loss, fetal death, preterm rupture of membranes and labour, and rhesus sensitization. Fetal skin and liver biopsy are now rarely required due to advances in molecular genetics, which allow diagnosis of many conditions from placental tissue without the need for histological examination of the affected organs.

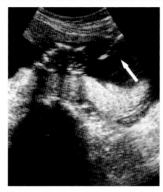

Fig 33 Ultrasound picture of amniocentesis (needle arrowed).

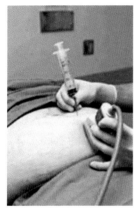

Fig 34 Amniocentesis: insertion of the needle under ultrasound guidance.

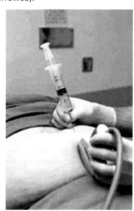

Fig 35 Amniocentesis: aspiration of liquor.

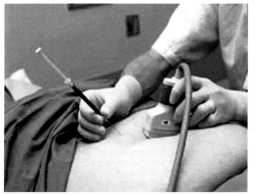

Fig 36 Fetal blood sampling.

Down syndrome (trisomy 21)

Incidence
Occurs in 1 in 700 live births and shows increasing incidence with older mothers (1 in 2000 at age 25, 1 in 365 at age 35 and 1 in 100 at age 40). Recurrence risk is usually determined by maternal age unless a rare parental balanced translocation exists.

Aetiology
Trisomy 21 in 94% of cases (Fig 37). Unbalanced translocation in 3% (half of which arise 'de novo') and mosaics in the remaining 3%.

Clinical features
Elevated risk of fetal loss, growth restriction, characteristic hypotonic facies (Fig 38), brachycephaly, single palmar creases, cardiac defects (40%), duodenal atresia, variable intellect, usually moderate learning difficulties.

Antenatal screening
Various methods exist, with differing sensitivities and positive predictive values. Universally available is the 'double test', performed at 15-19 weeks on maternal blood. Lower than average levels of α-fetoprotein and higher levels of hCG confer a higher risk. Women with a risk greater than 1 in 250 calculated on the basis of their age and these markers are offered a diagnostic test (see below). The 'triple' and 'quadruple' tests add in unconjugated estriol and inhibin to the assay, improving sensitivity of detection. More recently, nuchal translucency scanning at 11-13 weeks combined with first trimester biochemical markers has proved to be a more-sensitive screening tool for Down syndrome (see Fig 29). Women over the age of 37, or those with previously abnormal pregnancies, are often offered direct access to diagnostic tests (amniocentesis or chorionic villus sampling).

Edward syndrome (trisomy 18)

Incidence
1 in 3000 live births; risk increases with maternal age.

Aetiology
Trisomy 18 (Fig 39).

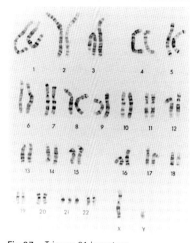

Fig 37   Trisomy 21 karyotype.

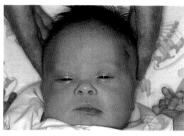

Fig 38   Baby with Down syndrome (trisomy 21).

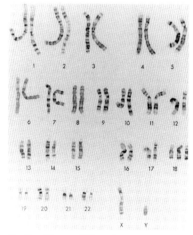

Fig 39   Trisomy 18 karyotype.

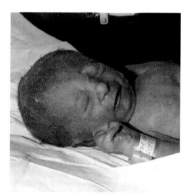

Fig 40   Baby with Edward syndrome.

Clinical features

Miscarriage/fetal death, growth restriction, severe learning defects, cardiac defects, hypoplastic lungs, flexion deformities, clenched fists with overlapping fingers (Fig 40), rocker-bottom feet, exomphalos, choroid plexus cysts, urogenital abnormalities. The majority die within a few months; less than 10% survive a year.

Patau syndrome (trisomy 13)

Incidence

Uncommon. Low recurrence risk. Risk increases with maternal age.

Aetiology

Trisomy 13 (Fig 41).

Clinical features

Miscarriage/fetal death, growth restriction, midline defects of the face, eyes and forebrain, holoprosencephaly, cleft lip and palate (Fig 42). Severe learning difficulties, deafness, rocker-bottom feet, polydactyly, congenital heart defects and cryptorchidism. Less than 20% survive the first year of life.

Turner syndrome (45,XO)

Incidence

Occurs in 1 in 5000 live births. Incidence is usually sporadic (i.e. not related to age or family history).

Aetiology

Single X chromosome.

Clinical features

Turner syndrome can present as miscarriage or fetal death, often with a cystic hygroma (Fig 43) or hydrops (Fig 44). Common features include growth restriction, neck webbing, broad chest with widely spaced nipples, low hairline and short neck and cubitus valgus. Coarctation of the aorta is found in 10% and a mild impairment of intellect is said to be characteristic.

Women with Turner syndrome are of short stature and experience failure of secondary sexual development. They have streak ovaries and are infertile. Oestrogen replacement is required.

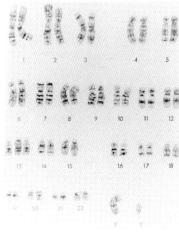

Fig 41 Trisomy 13 karyotype.

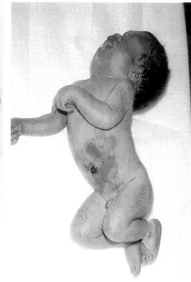

Fig 42 Newborn with Patau syndrome (trisomy 13).

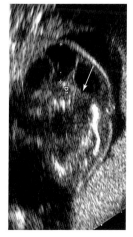

Fig 43 Ultrasound showing a cystic hygroma.

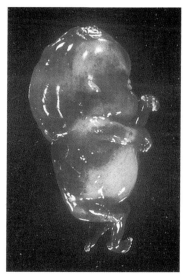

Fig 44 Fetus with Turner syndrome (45,XO).

Fetal imaging

Ultrasound

General
The majority of pregnant women in the UK have a routine scan in the first half of pregnancy.

Principles
All ultrasound machines work on the same basic principle. A probe is applied to the maternal abdomen or into the vagina, using a film of gel to ensure good contact.

The identification of structures in the ultrasound beam occurs by the same principle as sonar or radar. Diagnostic imaging uses a 1 ms pulse of ultrasound (usually 3.5 mHz) followed by a 1 ms gap for detection of the returning sound wave. By sequencing the firing of the transmitters in rapid succession, a real-time image is obtained (Fig 45).

By incorporating a mechanism for detecting blood flow by Doppler ultrasound it is possible to obtain a real-time image with a colour picture of blood flow (Fig 46).

More recent advances in technology have resulted in three-dimensional ultrasound images. These are useful in clarifying the detail of subtle surface abnormalities (e.g. facial clefts).

Applications
Determination of fetal viability and diagnosis of fetal abnormality, ectopic pregnancy, multiple pregnancy and trophoblastic disease. In the first half of pregnancy, it is used to assess gestational age; in the latter half of pregnancy for determining placental site and fetal presentation, documenting fetal growth and behaviour and measuring liquor volume. It is a mandatory adjunct for invasive procedures such as amniocentesis.

Other methods of fetal imaging

Fetoscopy (direct endoscopy) is invasive, risky and reserved for specific indications (e.g. laser ablation of placental vessels in the twin–twin transfusion syndrome). Fetal MRI is becoming increasingly popular in providing a more detailed assessment of central nervous system abnormalities (Fig 47).

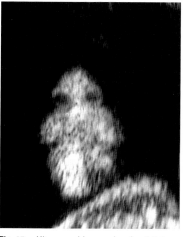

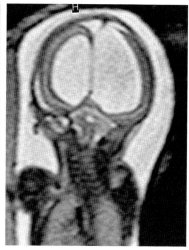

Fig 45 Ultrasound image showing fetal face (nostrils, lips and chin).

Fig 47 Fetal MRI showing ventriculomegaly.

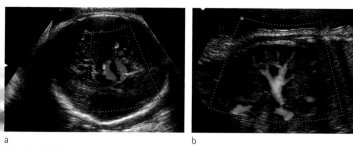

a   b

Fig 46 (a) Ultrasound using colour Doppler to demonstrate blood flow through the heart. (b) Power Doppler showing renal vascular anatomy.

Congenital abnormalities

Neural tube defects (NTD)

Types
Spina bifida (meningomyelocele, meningocele), anencephaly, encephalocele.

Incidence
Overall UK occurrence is about 1 in 1000, but there is geographical variation. In the UK, the incidence in registered births has fallen by 90% over the past two decades due to antenatal screening programmes (see below) and termination of affected pregnancies.

Aetiology
Combination of genetic factors and folic acid deficiency.

Prevention
Women with no personal or family history of NTD should take 400 μg of folic acid for at least 2 months preconceptually and to the end of the first trimester. Women with a previous or family history, or taking folate antagonists (e.g. anticonvulsants), should take 5 mg of folic acid in the periconceptual period.

Antenatal screening
Women are offered serum α-fetoprotein (AFP) screening at 16–18 weeks. A value of less than 2.3–2.5 times the population median indicates a low risk of NTD. A raised value makes NTD more likely, but other causes include fetal abdominal wall defects, multiple pregnancy, incorrect gestational age and bleeding in pregnancy. When the AFP value is raised, a detailed scan is undertaken (Fig 48). MRI can be used to further evaluate difficult cases (Fig 49).

Clinical features
- *Spina bifida*: a fluid-filled sac often containing neural tissue and an underlying defect of the spinal arch; 94% of cases are lumbosacral (Fig 50). The degree of handicap varies and can include paralysis of the lower limb, urinary and fecal incontinence, limb deformities, hip dislocations, urinary infections and hydrocephalus (70%).
- *Anencephaly*: absence of the forebrain and skull vault, facial distortion (Fig 51). It is incompatible with life.
- *Encephalocele*: herniation of the meninges and brain through the skull (usually occipital) (Fig 52).

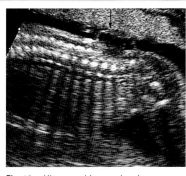

Fig 48 Ultrasound image showing lumbosacral meningocele (spina bifida).

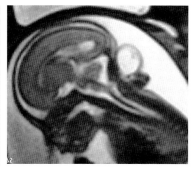

Fig 49 MRI of cervical meningocele.

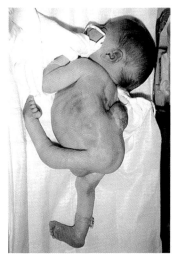

Fig 50 Newborn with spina bifida.

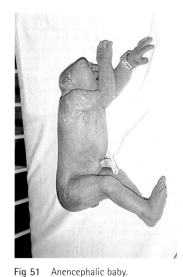

Fig 51 Anencephalic baby.

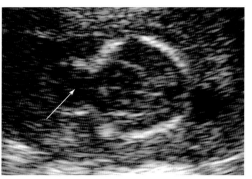

Fig 52 Ultrasound image of occipital encephalocele.

Skull/brain defects

Ventriculomegaly/hydrocephalus

Definition
Ventriculomegaly is enlargement of the cerebral ventricles with excessive intraventricular cerebrospinal fluid (Fig 53). If this causes enlargement of the skull it is known as hydrocephalus (Fig 54).

Aetiology
May occur in isolation or be secondary to aqueduct stenosis, intraventricular haemorrhage, fetal viral infection (e.g. cytomegalovirus) or neural tube defects. It is also associated with aneuploidy. Diagnosis is made by a combination of ultrasound with other investigations (e.g. viral studies, karyotyping). It should not be confused with conditions such as holoprosencephaly or porencephaly (Fig 55).

MRI may be helpful in clarifying the abnormality.

Prognosis
This varies and can be difficult to predict antenatally. Poor prognostic factors include the presence of other anomalies, severe ventriculomegaly with cortical thinning, and an accelerating rate of growth of the skull.

Ventricular shunts may be required after birth and even then the child may be irreversibly handicapped. Mild cases of ventriculomegaly detected antenatally may have a normal outcome. The degree of ventriculomegaly does not closely match outcome, however. If there is an underlying named major abnormality (such as NTD or aneuploidy), giving a prognosis is somewhat easier.

Microcephaly

Definition
A head circumference 3 standard deviations or more below the mean.

Aetiology
Often unknown, but may be familial. Pathological causes include congenital viral infections (e.g. rubella), inborn errors of metabolism, maternal phenylketonuria and many genetic malformation syndromes. Prognosis depends on the cause.

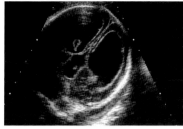

Fig 53 Coronal ultrasound scan showing ventriculomegaly.

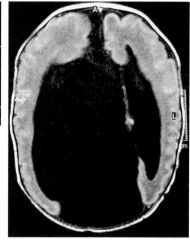

Fig 55 Fetal MRI showing porencephaly

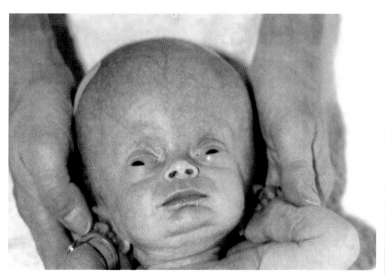

Fig 54 Baby with hydrocephalus.

Abdominal wall defects

Gastroschisis and exomphalos

Pathology
Uncommon. Failure of rotation and re-entry of gut into abdominal cavity during fetal development. Gastroschisis is possibly linked to environmental toxins; exomphalos is associated with aneuploidy.

Features
Both gastroschisis and exomphalos are associated with elevated maternal serum AFP and are diagnosed by ultrasound.

- *Gastroschisis*: defect of the abdominal wall separate from the insertion of the umbilical cord (Figs 56, 57). The abdominal viscera herniate and the peritoneal covering is lost. Usually an isolated defect.
- *Exomphalos*: herniation of the abdominal viscera through a defect at the umbilicus (Figs 58, 59). Usually the peritoneal covering is preserved and the umbilical cord is inserted on to the sac. Other congenital abnormalities are common (cardiac, bowel and chromosomal). Karyotyping by placental biopsy or blood sampling is advisable.

Management
Termination may be chosen if there are other anomalies or an abnormal karyotype. Otherwise, surgical closure is undertaken as soon as possible after birth. The neonate is at risk of hypothermia and/or dehydration. The operation may have to be a two-stage procedure, with the abdominal contents initially being enclosed in a temporary artificial sac. Mode of delivery does not influence the prognosis.

Prune belly syndrome

Aetiology
Uncommon, with only sporadic occurrence. Probably results from the in utero decompression of a massively enlarged bladder secondary to urethral obstruction.

Features
Deficient abdominal wall musculature, giving a rugose prune belly appearance. Undescended testes and renal anomalies are usually found and the latter determine outcome. If non-lethal, the abdominal wall is reconstructed in infancy.

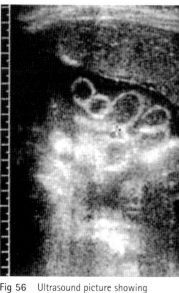

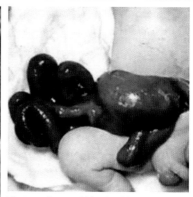

Fig 57 Gastroschisis after birth.

Fig 56 Ultrasound picture showing gastroschisis (loops of bowel floating free in amniotic cavity).

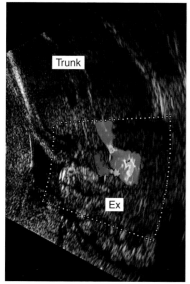

Trunk

Ex

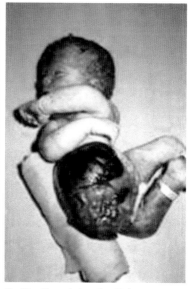

Fig 58 Ultrasound image showing exomphalos (Ex).

Fig 59 Exomphalos after birth.

Renal tract anomalies

Potter sequence

Incidence
1 in 3000 live births.

Aetiology
Caused by conditions producing oligohydramnios (e.g. renal agenesis—cause of original Potter syndrome), dysplastic kidneys, polycystic kidneys, urinary obstruction and chronic leakage of amniotic fluid.

Clinical features
Oligohydramnios, fetal growth restriction and fetal deformation. Low-set ears (Fig 60), compression abnormalities with limb flexion contractures, and hypoplastic lungs. Renal failure with urogenital causes.

Prognosis
Death is normally due to respiratory failure (pulmonary hypoplasia) soon after birth.

Urinary obstruction

Aetiology
May occur at the level of the pelvi-ureteric or vesico-ureteric junctions or the urethra (usually in males: posterior urethral valves).

Features
Hydronephrosis (Fig 61) or renal dysplasia may result. Severe bilateral disease will cause oligohydramnios and lung hypoplasia. A grossly distended bladder may occur with posterior urethral valves (Fig 62).

Management
Normal liquor volumes indicate some degree of renal function. Close postnatal follow-up is vital, however, and outcome is not well correlated with antenatal scan findings. Pregnancies with severe oligohydramnios are often terminated. Posterior urethral valves can be treated in utero by vesico-amniotic drain insertion, after careful case selection.

Ectopia vesicae

Features
Wide separation of pubic symphysis with ventral herniation of the bladder and exposure of bladder mucosa (Fig 63). Surgical correction is possible but incontinence is common.

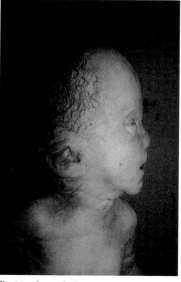

Fig 60 Potter facies.

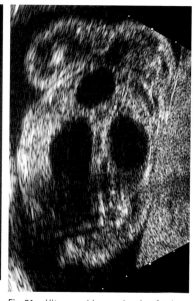

Fig 61 Ultrasound image showing fetal hydronephrosis and distended bladder.

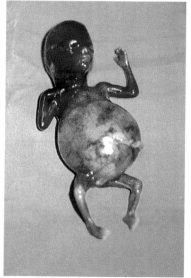

Fig 62 Fetus with posterior urethral valves and massive bladder distension.

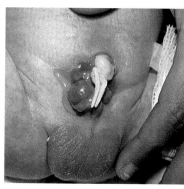

Fig 63 Ectopia vesicae.

Skeletal abnormalities

Osteogenesis imperfecta

Incidence
Rare (1 in 50 000 live births).

Aetiology
Mostly due to type I collagen abnormalities. Lethal forms result from new dominant mutations. Dominant inheritance is demonstrated in less severe forms.

Features
Types I-IV. Excessive tendency to antenatal and postnatal fractures which can be extremely deforming and disabling. Abnormal dentition and hearing loss may occur. Highly variable prognosis depending on type.

Diagnosis
The long bones are seen to be deformed and shortened on ultrasound and are poorly mineralized (as is the skull) with multiple fractures (Figs 64, 65). Rib involvement may cause respiratory compromise.

Short-limbed dwarfism

Incidence
Achondroplasia is the most common (10 in 10 000 live births).

Aetiology
New autosomal-dominant mutations in the fibroblast growth factor receptor-3 gene are responsible for most cases of achondroplasia and the more severe thanatophoric dwarfism (Fig 66). Mutations in the diastrophic dysplasia sulphate transporter gene cause achondrogenesis and diastrophic dysplasia. Campomelic dysplasia results from SOX-9 mutations.

Features
Each has its own pattern of abnormalities, but may include short limbs, large head, prominent forehead, narrow chest, poor ossification, polydactyly and facial clefting. Prognosis varies from good (achondroplasia) to lethal (e.g. thanatophoric dysplasia).

Limb reduction deformities

Causes include genetic syndromes, chorionic villus sampling earlier than 10 weeks, environmental toxins (e.g. thalidomide) and amniotic bands (Fig 67), in which clefting, encephalocele and gastroschisis may also occur.

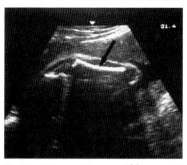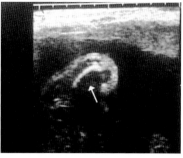

Fig 64   Ultrasound images of (a) a normal fetal femur, (b) an abnormal femur (shortening and bowing) (arrowed).

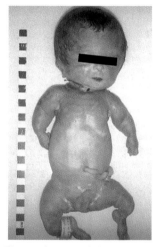

Fig 65   Osteogenesis imperfecta.

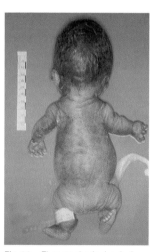

Fig 66   Thanatophoric dysplasia.

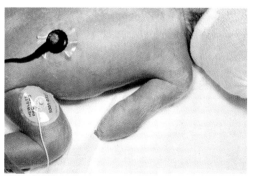

Fig 67   Distal limb amputation caused by amniotic bands.

Gastrointestinal anomalies

Diaphragmatic hernia

Incidence
1 in 1500 live births.

Aetiology
Failure of fusion or muscularization of the anterior and posterior leaves of the diaphragm allows abdominal contents to protrude into the chest (Fig 68). Often associated with aneuploidy, multiple malformation syndromes and cardiac defects.

Diagnosis
Ultrasound will normally demonstrate abdominal contents (liver or bowel) in the chest with displacement of the heart (Fig 69). Offer karyotyping and look for other anomalies.

Prognosis
The outcome is determined by the degree of pulmonary hypoplasia and the presence of other abnormalities. The overall survival rate is 70%.

Tracheo-oesophageal fistula

Incidence
1 in 3000 live births.

Aetiology
The oesophagus ends as a blind pouch. Varying degrees of pathological communication are found with the trachea, bronchi or lower oesophagus. Associated with other anomalies in 60% of cases.

Features
Polyhydramnios in 60% of cases. Absence of stomach bubble on ultrasound is an unreliable diagnostic sign as a fistula is present in 90%. The baby should not be fed until a gastric tube has been passed to test for gastric acid.

Intestinal obstruction

Polyhydramnios is common with small bowel obstruction. Ultrasound may show a 'double bubble' (Fig 70) with duodenal atresia (the first bubble is the stomach, the second bubble is the distended proximal duodenum—a marker for trisomy 21) and a 'triple bubble' with jejunal atresia.

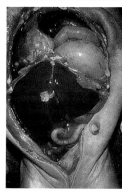

Fig 68 Postmortem of diaphragmatic hernia showing bowel in chest pushing the heart to the right.

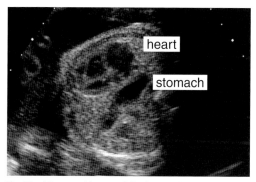

Fig 69 Ultrasound image of diaphragmatic hernia (stomach lies in the thorax, alongside the heart).

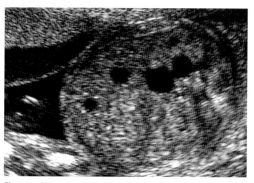

Fig 70 Ultrasound scan showing 'double bubble' of duodenal atresia.

Aetiology
Five allelic pairs of genes determine rhesus groups (C, c, D, E, e). The principal rhesus blood group is determined by the D locus. Rhesus (Rh) disease occurs when a Rh-negative mother has Rh antibodies and a Rh-positive baby. The antibodies cross the placenta and cause fetal haemolysis (anaemia, jaundice) and, in the extreme, cardiac failure and hydrops fetalis (Fig 71) and death. Rarely, Kell or Duffy antibodies can produce a similar severe disease. Less severe disease can be produced by antibodies to the C or E loci, A or B antigens.

Sensitization
Occurs when red blood cells from a Rh-positive fetus/baby enter the circulation of a Rh-negative woman (at delivery, abortion, placental bleeding, amniocentesis, chorionic villus sampling, external cephalic version, or spontaneously).

Prevention
By administration of anti-D immunoglobulin to Rh-negative mothers at potentially sensitizing events, or routinely at 28 and 34 weeks (depending on local policy).

Detection
Unsensitized Rh-negative women are screened for antibodies during pregnancy.

Assessment
The severity of disease may be assessed by amniotic fluid optical density difference at 450 nm (Fig 72), fetal blood sampling for fetal haemoglobin or non-invasively by measuring middle cerebral artery blood flow velocities (Fig 73). Hydrops on ultrasound is a late feature.

Intervention
Mild or moderate disease demands less frequent testing and delivery at term. More severe disease necessitates invasive testing and intrauterine transfusion of blood, often every 2-3 weeks. Intravenous immunoglobulins have been tried for severe disease at gestations too early for fetal blood transfusion.

Postnatal care
Cord blood is taken for haemoglobin, Coombs' test and bilirubin levels. Jaundice should be treated by phototherapy in mild cases and exchange transfusions in the more severe, to prevent kernicterus.

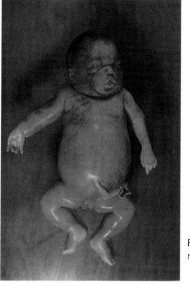

Fig 71   Hydrops fetalis secondary to rhesus disease.

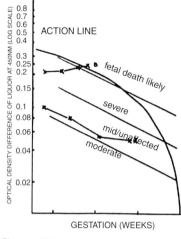

Fig 72   Liley curve with examples of moderate (a) and severe (b) disease.

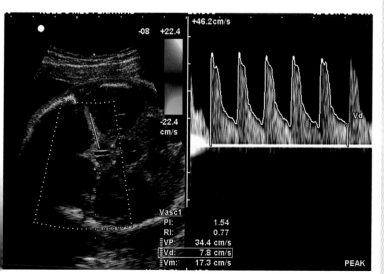

Fig 73   Doppler ultrasound of the middle cerebral artery.

Diagnosis
Fluid accumulation in skin (oedema) (Fig 74), abdomen (ascites) (Fig 75) or chest (pleural or pericardial effusions) (Fig 76), secondary to causes other than isoimmunization against red blood cell antigens.

Aetiology
- Anaemia: by haemolysis (red cell enzyme defects, homozygous α-thalassaemia), haemorrhage (twin–twin transfusion, fetomaternal haemorrhage), marrow infiltration (Gaucher disease) or parvovirus (B19) disease.
- Cardiac failure: arrhythmias, cardiac anomalies, cardiac tumour, or arteriovenous shunts (fetal or placental).
- Hypoproteinaemia: congenital nephrotic syndrome, hepatic enzyme defects.
- Obstructed venous return: neuroblastoma, cystic adenomatous malformation of lung, ovarian cysts, retroperitoneal fibrosis.
- Miscellaneous: congenital infection (parvovirus B19, cytomegalovirus, syphilis), chromosomal anomaly (e.g. Turner syndrome), skeletal dysplasias, chylo/hydrothorax, inborn errors of metabolism, neurological disorders.

Management
Once fetal hydrops has been noted, the cause should be identified, if possible, by a combination of ultrasound, maternal blood tests and fetal invasive testing. Even if a cause is found (80%), treatment may not be possible. Treatable causes include fetal anaemia (with intrauterine transfusion), fetal cardiac arrhythmia (with maternal administration of digoxin or flecainide) and pleural effusions (with insertion of pleuroamniotic shunts), which are occasionally the cause of more widespread oedema. Overall survival is about 25%.

Clinical features
The prognosis is improved by correction of the hydrops antenatally where possible. At delivery, a baby born with unresolved hydrops may be pale and suffer from congestive heart failure or severe respiratory distress due to pulmonary oedema or pulmonary hypoplasia with pleural effusions (Fig 77).

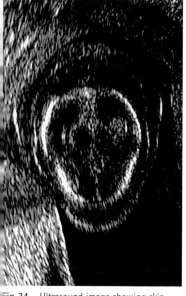

Fig 74 Ultrasound image showing skin oedema.

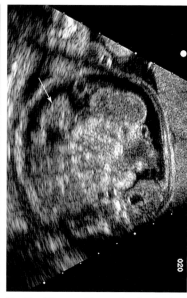

Fig 75 Ultrasound image showing fetal ascites.

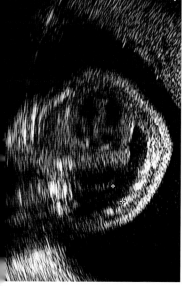

Fig 76 Ultrasound image showing a fetal pleural effusion.

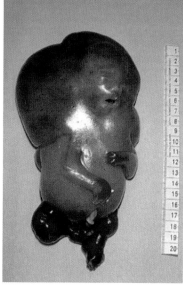

Fig 77 Dead hydropic baby.

Anaemia

Definition
The haemoglobin concentration varies with gestation. The lower limit of normal is 11 g/dL in the first trimester and 10.5 g/dL after 28 weeks.

Aetiology
Physiological (due to haemodilution) (Fig 78), iron deficiency (hypochromic, microcytic, low serum ferritin) (Fig 79) or folate deficiency (hyperchromic macrocytic, low red cell folate) (Fig 80). Vitamin B_{12} deficiency, infection, haemoglobinopathies and other causes are uncommon.

Prophylaxis
In some women, the daily iron requirement cannot be met by the diet. For such mothers, supplementation with iron (100 mg elemental iron per day), often with folic acid (300 mg/day), is recommended. The use of iron and folate supplements for all mothers is controversial in the prevention of anaemia; however, daily intake of folic acid of 400 µg periconceptually is recommended to prevent neural tube defects (see Ch 8).

Investigations
Once the diagnosis has been made, other investigations include red cell indices (mean corpuscular volume, mean corpuscular haemoglobin concentration), reticulocyte count, film, serum ferritin, red cell folate and serum vitamin B_{12} concentrations, and electrophoresis if a haemoglobinopathy is suspected.

Treatment
Depends on the cause. Mild physiological anaemia requires no treatment. Iron and/or folate deficiency can be treated with oral iron and folic acid together, although oral iron is often poorly tolerated (gastrointestinal disturbance). Parenteral iron can cause anaphylaxis (rashes, arthralgia, angioneurotic oedema) and should only be given when all oral preparations have been unsuccessful, and in hospital. Oral folic acid should be given with parenteral iron because of the stimulus to haemopoiesis. Blood transfusion in pregnancy should be a rare event (e.g. with symptomatic severe anemia).

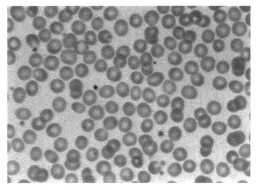

Fig 78   Normal blood film.

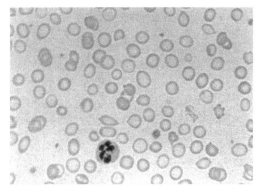

Fig 79   Blood film showing iron deficiency (hypochromia and microcytosis).

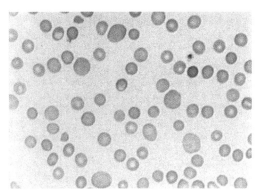

Fig 80   Blood film showing folate deficiency (macrocytosis).

Hypertension

Definition
A sustained absolute systolic BP of 140 mmHg or a diastolic BP of 90 mm Hg on more than one occasion at least 4 h apart. An alternative definition is a sustained rise of systolic BP by 30 mmHg and/or diastolic BP by 15 mmHg over booking values. This latter definition correlates less well with perinatal morbidity. Hypertension caused by pregnancy does not usually occur until after 20 weeks.

Examination
Semirecumbent/sitting relaxed mother, upper arm level with heart (Fig 81) and sphygmomanometer (larger cuff with obese women) (Fig 82). Diastolic BP is taken as the point at which the pulse can no longer be heard (Korotkoff phase V) and is more closely related to intra-arterial pressure than Korotkoff phase IV (muffling of the pulse). Different equipment (Fig 83) may produce significantly different values.

Classification
- Pregnancy-induced hypertension alone.
- Pregnancy-induced hypertension with proteinuria (pre-eclampsia).
- Pre-existing hypertension.
- Pre-existing hypertension with added pre-eclampsia.

Pre-existing hypertension

Aetiology
Mostly essential hypertension. Other diagnoses include renal pathology (multicystic/polycystic kidney disease, renal artery stenosis), endocrinopathies (Cushing syndrome/disease, Conn syndrome, phaeochromocytoma), connective tissue disorders, aortic coarctation, drugs (oral contraceptives, steroids).

Management
Change unsuitable antihypertensives (e.g. atenolol, diuretics and ACE inhibitors) where possible to medications safe for use in pregnancy (labetalol, methyldopa, nifedipine).

Serial scanning for evidence of placental disease and maternal monitoring for superimposed pre-eclampsia.

Pregnancies complicated by moderate-to-severe hypertension are usually induced at 38 weeks, if not sooner.

Pregnancy-

Management

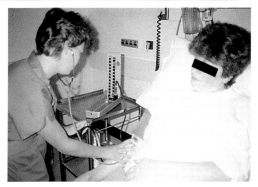

Fig 81   Measuring blood pressure.

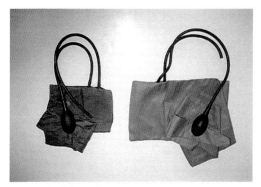

Fig 82   Cuff size variation.

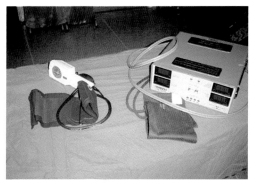

Fig 83   Equipment variation.

induced hypertension (without proteinuria)

Close fetal and maternal surveillance for evidence of pre-eclampsia or placental insufficiency. When the isolated hypertension is mild (<160/100 mmHg), early induction is not usually necessary. These pregnancies are not usually complicated by fetal growth restriction or increased maternal/perinatal morbidity or mortality.

Pre-eclampsia

Definition
Hypertension associated with significant proteinuria (>0.3 g per 24-h urine collection) in the absence of a urinary tract infection.

Aetiology
Condition peculiar to pregnancy of unknown aetiology, associated with multisystem endothelial damage and placental hypoperfusion. Occurs in 5% of all pregnancies. Risk factors: primigravidity, previous pre-eclampsia, family history, pre-existing hypertension, migraine, diabetes, connective tissue disorders, antiphospholipid syndrome, any condition associated with a large placenta (multiple pregnancy, hydatidiform mole, hydrops).

Clinical features
Characterized by hypertension, proteinuria, renal impairment, fluid retention and fetal growth restriction. Acute complications include eclampsia (secondary to cerebral oedema and vasospasm) (Fig 84), disseminated intravascular coagulation (Fig 85), liver capsule distension (Fig 86), pulmonary oedema (Fig 87) and abruption (Fig 127).

Symptoms include headache, visual disturbances and epigastric pain. Marked oedema, brisk reflexes, clonus and upper abdominal tenderness may be found on examination.

Management
Resolution of pre-eclampsia comes only with delivery. If very preterm (less than 34 weeks), close fetal and maternal monitoring as an inpatient is indicated. Maternal steroids should be given as preterm delivery may be necessary. Antihypertensives and anticonvulsants (magnesium sulphate) should be considered.

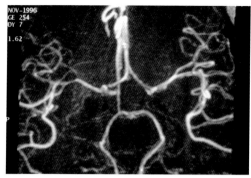

Fig 84   MRI of pre-eclamptic brain.

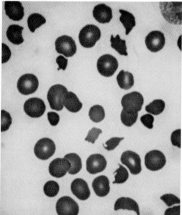

Fig 85   Blood film showing haemolysis.

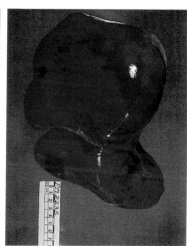

Fig 86   Subcapsular hepatic haemorrhage.

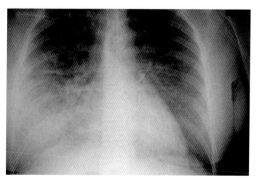

Fig 87   Chest X-ray showing pulmonary oedema.

Diabetes mellitus (DM)

Definition
Inadequate blood sugar control due either to a deficiency in production of insulin (type I) or to a state of insulin resistance (type II and gestational diabetes mellitus). Diagnosed by an oral glucose tolerance test (OGTT).

Pre-existing DM

Maternal risks   Increased insulin requirement, hypoglycaemic episodes, deterioration of retinopathy, pre-eclampsia and traumatic labour/caesarean section.

Fetal risks   Increased risk of congenital malformations (especially cardiac, musculoskeletal, neural tube defect) (Fig 88), macrosomia (Fig 89), polyhydramnios, fetal death, traumatic delivery (e.g. shoulder dystocia and Erb's palsy) (Fig 90), respiratory distress, hypoglycaemia and jaundice.

Management

Prepregnancy   High-dose folic acid and improved blood glucose control reduce the risk of congenital anomalies.

Antenatal   Close control of blood glucose (Fig 91). Aim for preprandial values of less than 6 mmol/L, and 2-h postprandial values less than 9.0 mmol/L. Insulin is substituted for oral hypoglycaemic agents. Regular checks of BP and optic fundi. Fetal screening for normality by ultrasound at 11-13 weeks (nuchal translucency) and 20 weeks. Later, regular scans for growth and well-being. Delivery at 38-40 weeks. Consider elective caesarean section for macrosomic babies. After delivery, insulin requirements fall.

Gestational DM

Diagnosis follows screening with random blood sugars and OGTT. This may be universal or include only those pregnant women with risk factors (glycosuria, family history of diabetes, unexplained stillbirth, previous macrosomia, maternal obesity, polyhydramnios).

Gestational DM may be managed by dietary changes alone. Insulin often required. Onset is usually after 24 weeks. Main risk is macrosomia and its complications.

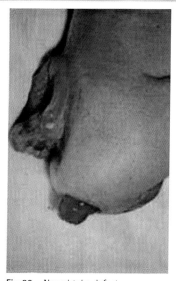

Fig 88   Neural tube defect.

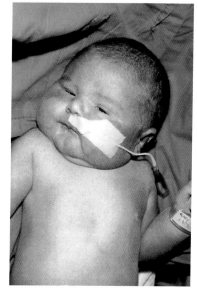

Fig 89   Macrosomia.

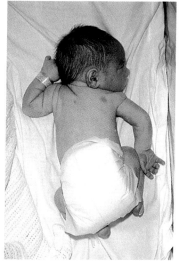

Fig 90   Erb's palsy.

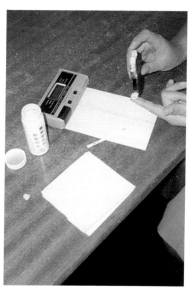

Fig 91   Frequent glucose testing to improve control.

Venous thromboembolic disease

Incidence
1 in 1500 pregnancies. It remains the leading cause of maternal mortality in the UK.

Aetiology
Pregnancy itself is a risk factor because of raised coagulation factors, reduced fibrinolysis and decreased levels of endogenous anticoagulants. These changes are most marked in the puerperium. Other risk factors include obesity, immobility, age (older than 35 years), dehydration, pre-eclampsia, inherited thrombophilias (e.g. antithrombin III deficiency), acquired thrombophilias (e.g. primary/secondary antiphospholipid syndrome) and operative delivery.

Clinical features
May present as a deep vein thrombosis (DVT; swollen, painful, warm lower leg and thigh) (Fig 92), pulmonary embolism (chest pain, haemoptysis, shortness of breath, tachycardia, collapse) or more rarely cerebral venous sinus thrombosis (headache, vomiting and reduced level of consciousness).

Diagnosis
A DVT is usually diagnosed by venous Doppler of the lower limbs. Pulmonary emboli are diagnosed by ventilation/perfusion scanning (Fig 93) or angiography. MRI is proving increasingly valuable in the diagnosis of all forms of thromboembolic disease in pregnancy (Fig 94).

Treatment
Traditional treatment of DVT and pulmonary embolism with intravenous unfractionated heparin is being replaced by subcutaneous injections of low molecular weight heparin. In rare cases, multiple pulmonary embolisms arising from a DVT can be prevented by insertion of a filter in the inferior vena cava (Fig 95). Anticoagulation during pregnancy increases the risks of antepartum and postpartum haemorrhage.

Prevention
Recognition of risk factors for thromboembolic disease is vital. Prophylaxis in the postpartum period, especially after caesarean section, is particularly important. Prophylaxis with low molecular weight heparin is often commenced antenatally and continued 6 weeks after delivery.

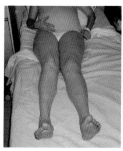

Fig 92   Left deep vein thrombosis.

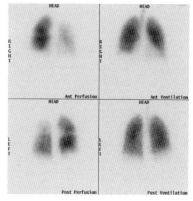

Fig 93   Scan showing ventilation/ perfusion mismatch due to pulmonary emboli.

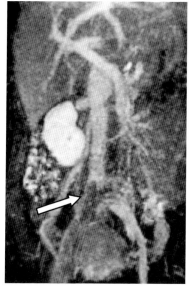

Fig 94   MRI of left ileofemoral thrombosis.

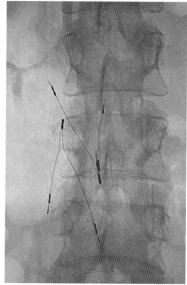

Fig 95   X-ray of inferior vena cava filter.

Sexually transmitted infections

Human immunodeficiency virus

Risk factors include intravenous substance abuse, African origin, partners with high-risk behaviours (e.g. bisexuality and unprotected intercourse). All pregnant women are offered HIV testing.

Risks
Without interventions, HIV is transmitted from mother to fetus in 15-25% of cases. Use of antiretroviral drugs through pregnancy, elective caesarean section and avoidance of breast feeding reduce this to less than 2%. HIV does not adversely affect pregnancy outcome in the absence of AIDS-defining illnesses (Fig 96).

Management
Jointly with an HIV physician. Antiretroviral drugs should be continued or commenced in those women not yet taking them. Screening and treatment of genital infections helps to reduce transmission, as does elective caesarean section and bottle-feeding. Regular CD4 counts. Extreme care in handling body fluids.

Genital herpes

Primary herpes infections (Fig 97) should be treated with 5 days of oral aciclovir; this should be recommenced in the late third trimester to prevent recurrences. Those presenting after 30 weeks' gestation should be delivered by caesarean section to prevent neonatal infection. The risk of this is almost negligible with secondary recurrences (due to passive immunity).

Group B streptococcus (GBS)

The most frequent cause of early onset neonatal sepsis, accounting for approximately 40 deaths per year in the UK. 20-30% of women have vaginal colonization (Fig 98). Those with previous neonatal infection should receive intrapartum antibiotic prophylaxis with penicillin. It is common practice for carriers without such a history to receive intrapartum antibiotics.

Others

Neisseria gonorrhoeae and *Chlamydia trachomatis* reside in the cervix. Intrapartum infection may cause conjunctivitis (Fig 99), arthritis, meningitis or generalized septicaemia. During pregnancy these infections are treated with penicillin and erythromycin, respectively.

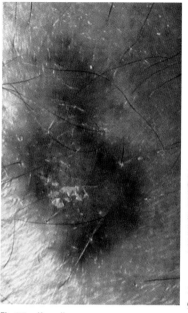

Fig 96 Kaposi's sarcoma.

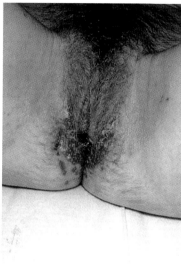

Fig 97 Herpes simplex infection of the genitalia.

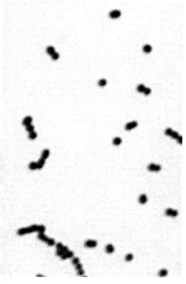

Fig 98 Gram stain of group B streptococcus.

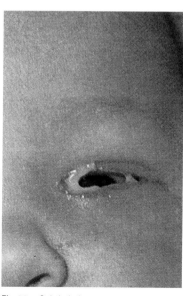

Fig 99 Ophthalmia neonatorum.

Dermatological problems

Pre-existing conditions

The skin manifestations of systemic lupus erythematosus (SLE), dermatomyositis and systemic sclerosis can recur in pregnancy, requiring treatment with oral steroids. Risk of fetal growth retardation and death is more common with all three conditions.

Eczema and psoriasis can worsen or improve in pregnancy.

Most dermatological treatments are safe during pregnancy, but the retinoids (psoriasis and acne), methotrexate (psoriasis), podophyllin (genital warts) and griseofulvin (fungal skin infections) should all be avoided.

Pregnancy-specific dermatoses

Specific dermatoses of pregnancy include polymorphic eruption (Fig 100) (0.75% incidence, erythematous edematous papules), pruritic folliculitis (Fig 101) (pruritic erythematous follicular papules), prurigo (Fig 102) (0.3% incidence, itchy excoriated papules) and pemphigoid ('herpes') gestationis (Fig 103) (1:50 000 incidence, recurrent condition associated with autoimmune conditions, pruritic urticarial papules, vesicles and bullae). The distribution is especially over abdomen and thighs. Treatment with oral antihistamines and topical 1% hydrocortisone is usually effective, although oral steroids may be required for pemphigoid gestationis.

Cholestasis of pregnancy

Obstetric cholestasis is itching secondary to pregnancy-related intrahepatic cholestasis (0.2% of pregnancies). There is a 40% recurrence risk. Typically presents in the third trimester with itching of palms of hands and soles of feet. There is no skin rash but excoriation marks may be present. Associated with an increased risk of prematurity and stillbirth. Diagnosis is by elevated serum bile acids and liver transaminases. The itching can sometimes be controlled with ursodeoxycholic acid. Delivery is the cure (normally electively at 37-38 weeks' gestation).

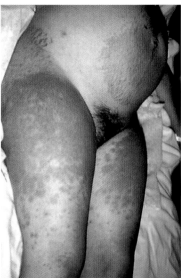

Fig 100   Polymorphic eruption of pregnancy.

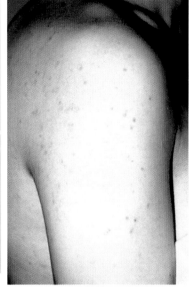

Fig 101   Pruritic folliculitis of pregnancy.

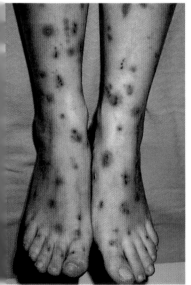

Fig 102   Prurigo of pregnancy.

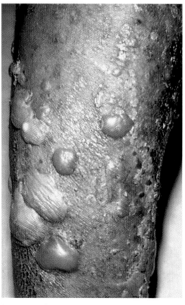

Fig 103   Pemphigoid gestationis.

Drugs and substance abuse

Prescribed drugs

Most drugs cross the placenta and are excreted in breast milk, but teratogenic effects have been confirmed for only a few (e.g. valproate, warfarin, methotrexate). However, drug therapy in the first trimester should be avoided if possible. Fetal growth and development can be affected later: e.g. tetracycline-induced staining of fetal teeth (Fig 104), antithyroid drugs producing fetal goitre (Fig 105). Drugs used in the third trimester may affect the newborn (e.g. narcotic analgesia causing neonatal depression). Drugs should only be prescribed when there are clear indications and benefits outweigh the risks.

Smoking

Maternal smoking reduces the mean birth weight by 200-300 g. Fetal growth restriction is limited by stopping smoking in the second half of pregnancy. Maternal smoking during pregnancy also increases the risk of preterm labour, preterm rupture of membranes, abruption and sudden infant death.

Alcohol

Consumption of more than 20 units of alcohol per week has been associated with intellectual impairment, alcohol-related birth defects and the fetal alcohol syndrome (mental retardation, growth retardation, characteristic facies with short palpebral fissures, hypoplastic nasal philtrum, and micrognathia) (Fig 106).

Substance abuse

Complications more common in women who abuse drugs during pregnancy include anaemia, premature membrane rupture, antepartum haemorrhage, preterm delivery, fetal growth restriction, birth asphyxia and perinatal death. They are also at risk of hepatitis B and HIV infection. Neonatal withdrawal symptoms may occur, the timing depending on the drug and its half-life.

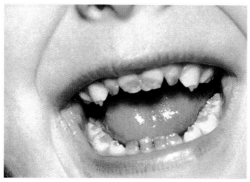

Fig 104   Tetracycline teeth.

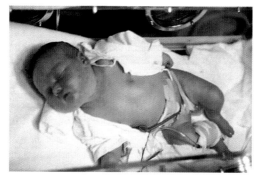

Fig 105   Neonatal goitre secondary to maternal antithyroid treatment.

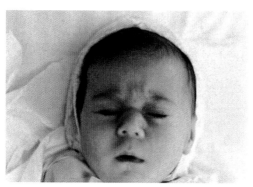

Fig 106   Fetal alcohol syndrome.

12 Fetal growth restriction

Incidence

Approximately 10% of all live-born babies and 30% of those weighing less than 2.5 kg suffer from intrauterine growth restriction (IUGR). They experience greater perinatal mortality and morbidity and have more developmental problems later in life.

Definition

IUGR is defined as 'failure of a fetus to achieve its genetic growth potential' (Fig 107). In practice, however, the diagnosis is not always easy as there are ethnic and geographical variations. Antenatal identification is usually based on ultrasound: failure of fetal biometric measurements to progress along an earlier centile within the normal population range, or marked asymmetry between the head circumference (Fig 108) and abdominal circumference (Fig 109). It is important to note that fetal size does not have to fall outside the normal range for this diagnosis to be made.

In normal growth, maximum velocity of linear growth occurs at 20 weeks, and of body weight at 34 weeks. At the end of pregnancy, physical constraints probably slow fetal growth. Control is influenced by genetic and hormonal factors and nutrient supply.

Causes

- *Intrinsic causes*: malformations, including chromosomal abnormalities (5-10%) and viral infections (2%).
- *Extrinsic causes*: uteroplacental vascular insufficiency (e.g. pre-eclampsia), cyanotic heart disease, maternal malnutrition if severe, smoking, alcohol, cocaine, medications (e.g. atenolol) and idiopathic causes (30%).

Risk factors

Short stature, previous small baby, low maternal weight (<45 kg) and body mass index, poor weight gain, multiple pregnancy, smoking, alcohol, raised α-fetoprotein and other conditions (see causes above).

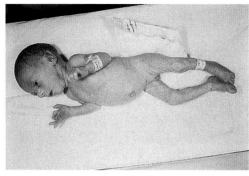

Fig 107   Growth-restricted newborn infant.

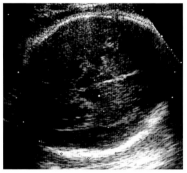

Fig 108   Head circumference measurement at ultrasound.

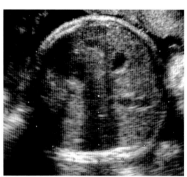

Fig 109   Abdominal circumference measurement at ultrasound.

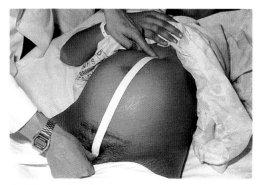

Fig 110   Fundal height measurement.

Diagnosis

Even with a high degree of clinical suspicion based on risk factors, 30-50% of growth-restricted fetuses remain undetected by clinical examination. Serial recording of symphysiofundal height improves the sensitivity of detection but is nevertheless poor (Fig 110). Multiple pregnancy, polyhydramnios, transverse lie and maternal obesity further reduce clinical detection rates. Ultrasound is the best method of diagnosing pathological fetal growth using serial measurements of head (HC) and abdominal (AC) circumferences.

Two patterns of IUGR are recognized:

- *Symmetrical/early*: usually due to intrinsic problems (e.g. congenital abnormality, viral infection). On ultrasound, both HC and AC measurements fall away from expected growth trajectories (Fig 111).
- *Asymmetrical/late*: usually due to extrinsic problems (e.g. pre-eclampsia, multiple pregnancy). On ultrasound, AC values fall away from expected growth trajectories but HC growth is mostly maintained (Fig 112).

Management

The growth-restricted fetus should be scanned for congenital abnormalities. Karyotyping by amniocentesis or chorionic villus sampling and viral studies should be considered in early-onset or symmetrical cases. Serial monitoring of fetal health is mandatory. The timing of elective delivery is determined by gestation and fetal health assessment. Consideration should be given to administering steroids in preterm cases. Doppler analysis of umbilical artery blood flow may be used to differentiate the normally grown small fetus from one with pathological growth due to uteroplacental disease.

Neonatal complications

Perinatal asphyxia, meconium aspiration, pulmonary haemorrhage, hypothermia, hypoglycaemia, polycythaemia and possibly prematurity and congenital abnormalities.

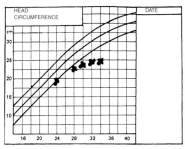

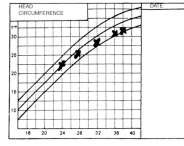

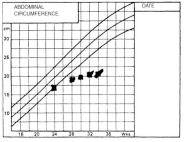

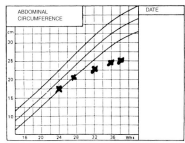

Fig 111 Symmetrical/early fetal growth restriction.

Fig 112 Asymmetrical/late fetal growth restriction.

13 > Antepartum fetal health assessment

Routine screening

In low-risk pregnancies this is limited to clinical assessment of fetal growth and the maternal perception of fetal movements/activity. The fetal heart is recorded routinely either by auscultation with a Pinard stethoscope (Fig 113) or with simple hand-held Doppler ultrasound (Fig 114). Recording of the fetal heart in this way is a limited assessment of fetal well-being. It is able to detect only whether the fetal heart is present, and whether the rate is normal at any given moment.

Pregnancies at risk

A pregnancy may be deemed 'high-risk' as a result of previous medical/obstetric history (e.g. maternal systemic lupus erythematosus, previous stillbirth) or because of events occurring during pregnancy (e.g. raised serum α-fetoprotein, recurrent antepartum haemorrhage, pregnancy-induced hypertension, ultrasonically diagnosed intrauterine growth restriction—IUGR). Serial ultrasound should be performed in such pregnancies for biometric parameters, estimation of liquor volume, fetal biophysical testing and possibly umbilical artery Doppler measurement. Non-stress fetal heart rate (FHR) monitoring also has a role in fetal antenatal assessment (Fig 115). The value of these monitoring techniques has not been established for certain conditions (e.g. diabetes, obstetric cholestasis).

Biophysical methods

The underlying principle is that the fetus exposed to a chronic insult (especially hypoxia) will have a depressed central nervous system (reduced heart-rate variability, movements, tone and breathing movements) and, if severe, depressed renal function (oligohydramnios). The tests used are the kick chart (daily record of maternally perceived movements), non-stress FHR recording and the biophysical profile (see below).

Cardio-tocography

There is a close association between an abnormal FHR pattern and an acutely asphyxiated fetus. The normal FHR trace at term is dependent on the state of the fetus. A mature fetus will be quiet for about 30% of the time

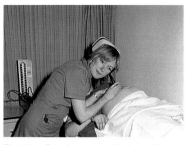

Fig 113 Fetal heart auscultation with a Pinard stethoscope.

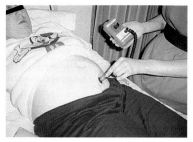

Fig 114 Fetal heart auscultation with hand-held Doppler.

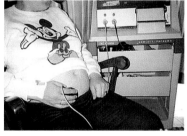

Fig 115 Fetal heart rate recording with cardiotocography.

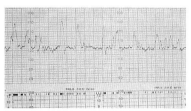

Fig 116 Reactive fetal heart rate recording at term.

(associated with little oscillation of the baseline and no accelerations) and active for about 70% of the time (wide oscillations of the baseline and many accelerations, i.e. rises in the FHR of 15 beats/min above the baseline lasting for at least 15 s) (Fig 116). A cardiotocogram (CTG) with accelerations, a baseline rate of between 110 and 160 beats/min and no decelerations is described as normal or 'reactive'. Cardiotocography is reliable at excluding asphyxia while it is being performed but offers little reassurance in the long term. It is most valuable for monitoring a fetus already known to be compromised and for intrapartum fetal monitoring.

Biophysical profile scoring (BPS)

A more comprehensive assessment of the fetus at risk of asphyxia is provided by the BPS, which records the presence of five biophysical variables: FHR pattern (non-stress test as above), fetal movements, fetal tone, fetal breathing and amniotic fluid volume. If four or five of these parameters are present in up to 30 min of recording, then the risk of terminal fetal asphyxia is low.

Amniotic fluid volume (AFV)

AFV can be measured by ultrasound using either maximum pool diameter (MPD) (range 20–80 mm) or amniotic fluid index (AFI; sum of four vertical pools of amniotic fluid measured in the four quadrants of the uterus) (Fig 117).

* *Oligohydramnios* (MPD <20 mm or AFI <3rd centile): can be due to ruptured membranes, fetal renal abnormality or fetal illness (e.g. severe IUGR).
* *Polyhydramnios* (MPD >80 mm or AFI >97th centile): can be due to a failure of fetal swallowing (e.g. tracheo-oesophageal atresia), excess urine production (e.g. infant of diabetic mother) or the twin–twin transfusion syndrome.

Doppler recording of umbilical artery blood flow

The absence of forward flow in diastole in the umbilical arteries of a small-for-dates fetus (Fig 118), or even reversed flow, is associated with an increased risk of perinatal death, birth asphyxia, need for preterm birth and necrotizing enterocolitis. This is the only test of fetal health with proven benefit from randomized trials. Changes in the blood flow patterns in other fetal blood vessels such as the ductus venosus (Fig 119) or middle cerebral artery (Fig 73) may help optimize decision-making regarding timing of delivery in severe early-onset IUGR.

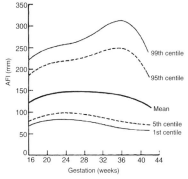

Fig 117 Amniotic fluid index (AFI) centile chart.

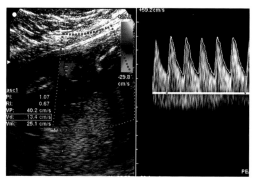

Fig 118 Umbilical artery Doppler blood flow recording.

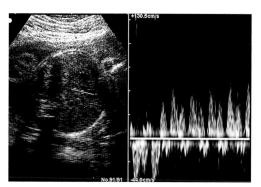

Fig 119 Blood flow recording from the ductus venosus.

Preterm birth

Definition
Delivery at less than 37 weeks' gestation.

Incidence
5-8% of all deliveries.

Causes
Risk factors for preterm labour include multiple gestation, antepartum haemorrhage, fetal abnormality, uterine abnormality, incompetent cervix, infection, preterm rupture of membranes (see below) and polyhydramnios. Preterm birth may be necessary because of pre-eclampsia, severe intrauterine growth restriction (IUGR), or deteriorating maternal health.

Management
Confirm the diagnosis of preterm labour by finding cervical change in association with regular uterine activity. Look for and treat any reversible causes. Use tocolysis (e.g. atosiban, ritodrine or nifedipine) if there are no contraindications. Give dexamethasone or betamethasone to reduce the incidence of respiratory distress syndrome (Fig 120).

Preterm rupture of membranes

Definition
Membrane rupture before uterine contractions at less than 37 weeks' gestation. 30% of preterm deliveries are preceded by preterm membrane rupture.

Diagnosis
Liquor at the introitus or in the vagina on speculum examination (Fig 121). The diagnosis can be difficult to make if loss of amniotic fluid is intermittent. Biochemical swab tests have been designed specifically for this purpose (Fig 122). Ultrasound scanning is not a sensitive test for this.

Consequences
Preterm labour and delivery, chorioamnionitis, postpartum endometritis and neonatal sepsis. Prolonged preterm rupture

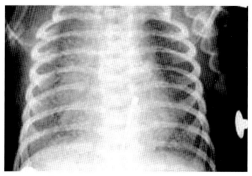

Fig 120 Neonatal chest X-ray showing the 'ground-glass' appearance of respiratory distress syndrome.

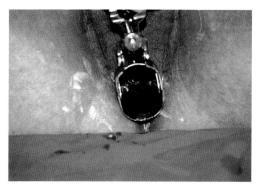

Fig 121 Liquor in the vagina seen via a sterile speculum.

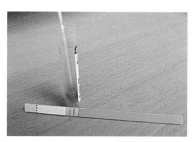

Fig 122 Biochemical swab testing for ruptured membranes.

of membranes from a very early gestation results in pulmonary hypoplasia, umbilical cord compression and postural deformities.

Management
Inpatient care is usually preferred but is not mandatory. A high degree of vigilance for infection is vital (pain, contractions, uterine tenderness, offensive discharge, maternal pyrexia, tachycardia, raised C-reactive protein, positive low vaginal swab) and vaginal examinations should be limited unless labour is suspected. For women between 24 and 34 weeks' gestation, empirical treatment with erythromycin prolongs the pregnancy and reduces infectious morbidity. Steroids are usually administered prior to 36 weeks to promote fetal lung maturation.

Delivery should be expedited at all gestations if infection is suspected. Only attempt to stop labour if it occurs within 48 h (provided steroids are given at presentation). For pregnancies extending beyond 34 weeks, an induction is usually organized at 36–38 weeks.

Consequences of preterm birth

Early neonatal complications include death, respiratory distress syndrome, intraventricular haemorrhage, periventricular leukomalacia (Fig 123), pulmonary haemorrhage, necrotizing enterocolitis (Fig 124), sepsis, hypothermia, poor feeding, jaundice, hypoglycaemia. Later complications include retinopathy, chronic lung disease and neurodevelopmental delay.

Prevention of preterm labour

Risk assessment
A risk assessment can be made on the basis of history (e.g. previous preterm birth, history of cone biopsy), specialized cervical swabs that detect fetal fibronectin, high vaginal swabs for bacteriology and cervical length scanning (Fig 125). A cervix shorter than 2.5 cm is significantly associated with an increased risk of preterm labour or rupture of membranes, particularly if cervical funneling is noted at the internal os.

Treatment
Women with bacterial vaginosis and a history of previous preterm birth may benefit from antibiotics. Those with cervical shortening and/or funnelling or with a history of cervical incompetence may benefit from a cervical suture.

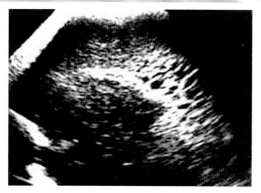

Fig 123 Ultrasound of neonatal brain showing periventricular leukomalacia.

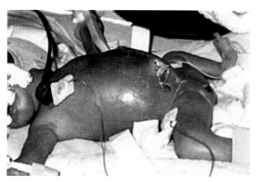

Fig 124 Neonate with necrotizing enterocolitis.

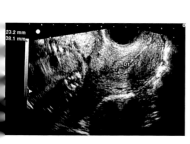

a

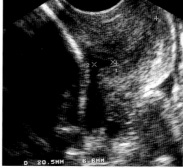

b

Fig 125 Transvaginal scans showing (a) a long (61.3 mm) closed cervix and (b) a short cervix (21.5 mm) with funnelling.

15 Antepartum haemorrhage

Definition

Bleeding from the genital tract from 24 weeks' gestation and before delivery of the baby.

Management

Assess blood loss and resuscitate. The fetal condition should be assessed. Establish cause. A vaginal examination should be avoided until the placental site is established with ultrasound. Vasa praevia and major abruption demand urgent delivery whereas placenta praevia can more often be managed conservatively with elective delivery later, usually by caesarean section.

Placenta praevia

Bleeding from a placenta encroaching into the lower uterine segment. Often painless or associated with contractions. Abnormal fetal lie/presentation common.

Graded as 'major' or 'minor' depending on whether or not the placental edge actually crosses the internal os.

Risk factors include previous caesarean section, multiple pregnancy and uterine anomaly.

Diagnosis is by ultrasound (Fig 126), MRI or examination in theatre.

Abruption

Bleeding from a normally situated placenta. Usually painful and associated with contractions or hypertonic, hard and tender uterus. The amount of blood passed vaginally can vary. It is unusual to see any bleeding on ultrasound. Cardiotocographic abnormalities and intrauterine fetal death or asphyxia are common. A retroplacental clot is often found at delivery (Fig 127) and a Kleihauer test may be positive (Fig 128), indicating fetomaternal transfusion of fetal red blood cells.

Vasa praevia

Bleeding from abnormally placed fetal vessel coursing through the membranes at the time of spontaneous or artificial membrane rupture. Often found with velamentous insertion or succenturiate lobe (Fig 129). The blood lost is from the fetal circulation and perinatal mortality rates are high.

Other causes

A 'show' at the onset of labor, cervical lesions (e.g. ectropion, cancer, cervicitis secondary to infection).

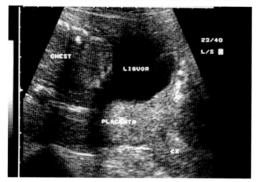

Fig 126   Ultrasound image showing placenta praevia (cx = cervix).

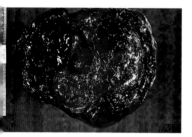

Fig 127   Abruption with visible retroplacental clot.

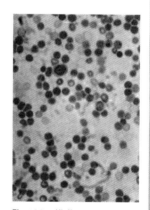

Fig 128   Kleihauer test.

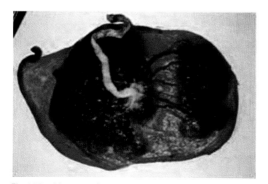

Fig 129   Vasa praevia.

General principles

Management

Everyone involved in the birth of a child should be concerned with the safety and health of the mother and baby and should strive to make the birth a satisfying experience for all concerned.

In many countries, overall conduct is the responsibility of a midwife alone or with reference to a general practitioner. An obstetrician is only involved if problems are present (e.g. fetal compromise, poor progress in labour, maternal disease). However, in other countries (e.g. the USA), the great majority of deliveries are conducted by obstetricians.

Monitoring

Labour should be a normal event, and management incorporates a programme of surveillance/monitoring that helps to detect deviation from this. There are three components of this monitoring, summarized on the partogram (one chart but displayed in three sections):

- *Fetal condition* (Fig 130). The fetal heart rate (FHR) is recorded either intermittently, every 15 min, or continuously by cardiotocogram (CTG). The colour of the liquor draining vaginally is recorded, and the degree of caput and/or molding judged from vaginal examinations performed every 4 h.
- *Progress of labour* (Fig 131). Record of the descent of the head (assessed abdominally in fifths, and vaginally in centimetres with respect to the ischial spines), the dilatation of the cervix on regular vaginal examinations, the strength and frequency of contractions, and drugs given to augment/induce labour.
- *Maternal condition* (Fig 132). General well-being, pulse and blood pressure are recorded every half-hour, temperature every 4 h. Fluid intake and urine output are recorded and the urine is also tested for glucose, protein and ketones. Any drugs given to the woman are also noted.

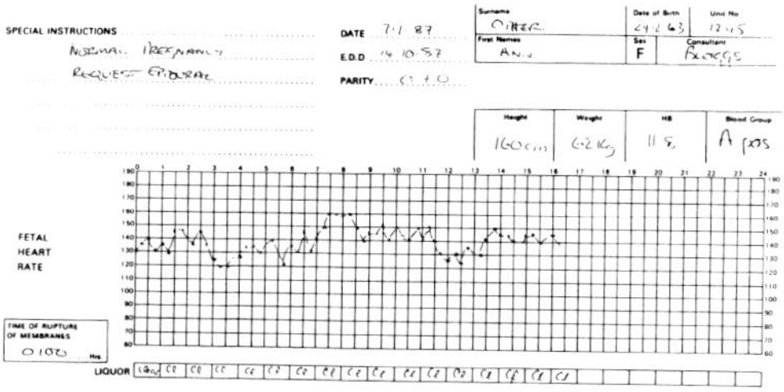

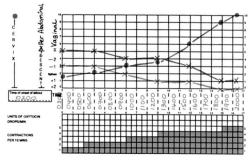

Fig 130   Partogram: fetal section.

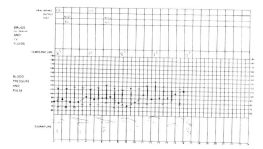

Fig 131   Partogram: progress section.

Fig 132   Partogram: maternal section.

The first stage

Definition
From the onset of labour to full dilatation of the cervix.

Diagnosis
The onset of labour is a retrospective diagnosis made when serial vaginal examinations show progressive cervical change (effacement and dilatation) in the presence of regular contractions. It is often associated with a 'show'— the passage vaginally of a blood-stained mucous plug from the cervix. Membrane rupture precedes labour in only about 10% of cases.

Phases
- *Latent phase*: from the onset of labour to when the cervix is about 3-4 cm dilated and fully effaced. Mean duration is 9 h in primigravidae and 5 h in multigravidae.
- *Active phase*: from the end of the latent phase to full dilatation. The mean duration is 5 h in primigravida and 2 h in multigravida. During this phase the cervix should dilate at least 1cm per hour and the presenting part should descend (Fig 133).

Poor progress
Two patterns of delay in first stage are recognized from the partogram. Primary dysfunctional labour (Fig 134) describes poor progress throughout the active phase. It is more common in primiparous women and is often caused by inefficient uterine activity and fetal malposition (e.g. occipitoposterior). Secondary arrest (Fig 135) occurs when previously good progress slows or comes to a halt. More commonly found with malpresentation (e.g. brow) or cephalopelvic disproportion, which occurs when the fetus is too large for the pelvis.

Management
A diagnosis should be made. If inefficient uterine activity is the cause, dehydration should be corrected and the membranes ruptured if still intact. Augmentation with oxytocin should be considered and can be monitored with an intrauterine pressure catheter (Fig 136). Caesarean section may be indicated for cephalopelvic disproportion or malpresentation.

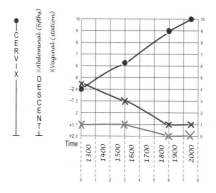

Fig 133   Partogram: normal progress.

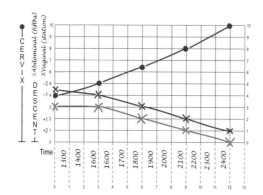

Fig 134   Partogram: slow progress.

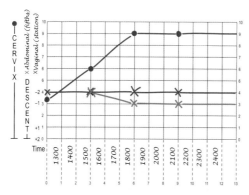

Fig 135   Partogram: secondary arrest.

Second stage

Definition
From full dilation of the cervix to delivery of the baby. Average duration is 40 min in primiparous women and 20 min in multiparae.

Phases
- *Propulsive/passive*: the presenting part is high and there is no desire to push.
- *Expulsive/active*: the presenting part is low and the mother wishes to push.

Management
The woman is usually encouraged to push when she feels the urge to 'bear down'. This reflex may be blocked in a woman with an epidural. Second stage should last no longer than 3 h and should be limited if there are concerns about maternal or fetal condition, with instrumental delivery if necessary. Women who have not given birth after an hour of active second stage should be carefully assessed. Augmentation with oxytocin may help, but assisted delivery may be more appropriate.

Crowning is said to occur as the introitus becomes maximally stretched (Fig 137). The left hand prevents too rapid a delivery and decompression of the fetal head. The right hand prevents uncontrolled tearing of the perineum. A hand is inserted to check for the presence of the cord around the baby's neck (Fig 138). If found, it is either clamped and cut or pulled over the head.

While the head is on the perineum it usually rotates to realign with the axis of the shoulders. The mother pushes again and, with the hands placed over the baby's parietal eminences, gentle traction is applied posteriorly to encourage the delivery of the anterior shoulder (Fig 139). Anterior traction is then applied, and the posterior shoulder and the body are delivered. An intramuscular injection of an oxytocic agent is given with the delivery of the anterior shoulder. Once the baby is delivered, the cord is double-clamped and cut (Fig 140). The baby is dried and wrapped and handed to the mother. The Apgar score is used to record the condition of the baby at birth.

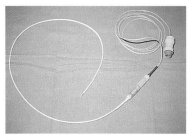

Fig 136   Intrauterine pressure catheter.

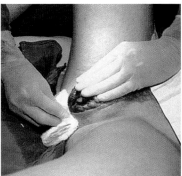

Fig 137   Crowning of the fetal head.

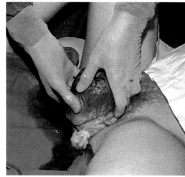

Fig 138   Checking for umbilical cord.

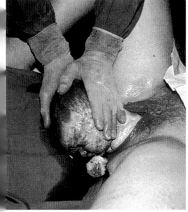

Fig 139   Delivery of the anterior shoulder.

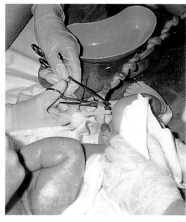

Fig 140   Clamping and cutting umbilical cord.

Third stage

Definition
From the birth of the baby to the delivery of the placenta.

Management
Active management is associated with a reduction in blood loss at delivery. It involves the administration of an oxytocic agent (e.g. intramuscular oxytocin 5 units with ergometrine 0.5 mg, or intramuscular oxytocin 10 units) with the delivery of the anterior shoulder, clamping and cutting the cord, and assisted delivery of the placenta once there are signs of separation: contraction of the uterus, a gush of blood (Fig 141) and descent/lengthening of the cord. The placenta and membranes are delivered by controlled cord traction (Figs 142, 143).

Physiological third stage uses no oxytocic agent or cord clamping and the placenta delivers spontaneously. It carries a higher incidence of primary postpartum haemorrhage.

Primary postpartum haemorrhage

Incidence
Occurs in 5% of births.

Definition
The loss of 500 mL of blood or more within 24 h of delivery.

Causes
Hypotonic uterus (caused by wholly or partially retained placenta, multiple pregnancy, large baby, polyhydramnios, lax uterus associated with high parity), trauma (e.g. uterine rupture, cervical or vaginal lacerations) and clotting disorders.

Management
Uterine atony is treated by intravenous oxytocics or intramuscular prostaglandins. An examination under anaesthesia may be necessary if the cause is uncertain. Special uterine sutures (B-Lynch) or intrauterine balloons may be used for uterine atony. Internal iliac artery ligation or hysterectomy may be necessary on rare occasions. A haematologist should be involved in major cases to advise on the use of blood products.

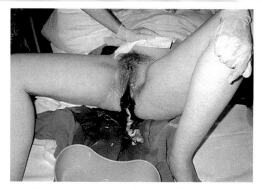

Fig 141   Blood flow and uterine contraction.

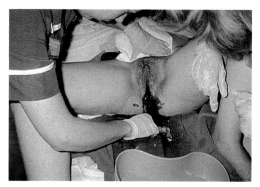

Fig 142   Controlled cord traction.

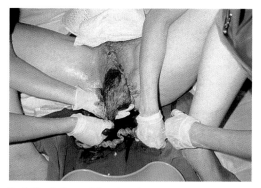

Fig 143   Delivery of the placenta.

Intrapartum fetal monitoring

Liquor

Normally the liquor is clear. Passage of meconium (Fig 144) may be due to hypoxia and is an indication for continuous FHR monitoring. Innocent causes are post-dates fetus and breech presentation. Meconium aspiration may occur and expert care is needed at birth to prevent this. Mild blood staining may be just a 'show'. Heavier bleeding may be due to placental abruption, placenta praevia or vasa praevia.

FHR monitoring

Aim
The detection of intrapartum hypoxia and acidosis. Fetal hypoxia causes a rise in pCO_2, and a metabolic acidosis secondary to an accumulation of lactate from anaerobic glycolysis. The fetal blood pH falls. This in turn causes FHR abnormalities. Many other less sinister factors have an impact on the FHR, and recognizing patterns associated with fetal compromise can be difficult. Estimation of fetal pH by fetal blood sampling is often necessary.

Routine
In low-risk pregnancies, the fetal heart is normally recorded intermittently every 15 min in first stage and after every contraction in second stage. The use of continuous FHR monitoring for all pregnancies should be discouraged.

Continuous FHR monitoring
This should be used in pregnancies with an increased risk of intrapartum hypoxia (e.g. fetal growth restriction, prematurity, breech presentation, multiple pregnancy, epidural analgesia, induced or augmented labour, diabetes, hypertension, bleeding, rhesus disease), auscultated FHR abnormalities or meconium staining.

It is performed using external Doppler ultrasound recording (Fig 145) or a fetal scalp electrode (Fig 146). Inherent risks of skin electrodes (scalp trauma and infection) make an external transducer preferable (provided a good-quality recording is obtained).

Cardio-tocography

Interpretation
Baseline rate   Normal at term is 110-160 beats/min. A low baseline (105-110 beats/min) may be normal if post-dates. Lower rates, especially if accompanied by other adverse features, may indicate hypoxia. Fetal tachycardia (baseline rate >160 beats/min) may be due to hypoxia or maternal pyrexia. A rise over the course of the labour, even if within normal limits, may also be important.

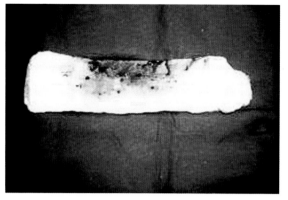

Fig 144   Meconium.

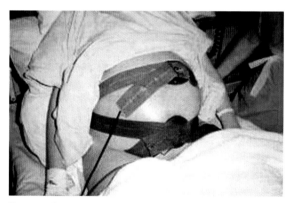

Fig 145   External cardiotocography.

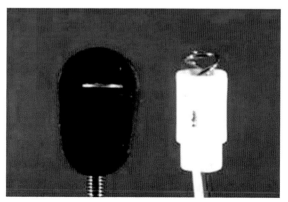

Fig 146   Fetal scalp electrodes.

Baseline variability   Normal is 5-25 beats/min. Reduced baseline variability may occur with fetal sleep states, hypoxia or maternal drug therapy (e.g. pethidine).

Accelerations   Defined as a rise in the FHR above the baseline of at least 15 beats/min, lasting at least 15 s. The presence of accelerations is a reliable sign of fetal well-being. A 'reactive' CTG (Fig 147) has two or more accelerations occurring in response to fetal movement.

Decelerations   Various types are recognized:
- *Early* (Fig 148): begins with contraction and returns to baseline by end of contraction; commonly due to change of pressure on fetal head (engagement, full dilation) (5% risk of low pH).
- *Variable* (Fig 149): variable in timing with respect to contraction, depth and duration; often due to cord compression (25% risk of low pH).
- *Late* (Fig 150): deceleration of FHR after the peak of a contraction; commonly due to placental insufficiency (50% risk of low pH).

Contractions   The frequency, but not the strength, of contractions can be determined by the CTG.

Classification
- *Normal*: the CTG has no abnormal features.
- *Suspicious*: one feature is abnormal; continued close observation is indicated.
- *Pathological*: more than one abnormal feature is present; the fetal condition needs to be investigated with fetal blood sampling (FBS). If this is not possible, then the baby should be delivered immediately.

Management of pathological CTG
The woman should be turned into a left lateral position to maximize uterine blood flow and placental oxygen transport. Some advocate giving oxygen by face mask. Any hypotension should be corrected swiftly with intravenous fluids (e.g. after an epidural has been sited) and an oxytocin infusion (if present) turned off. Acute and irreversible causes of CTG abnormalities (e.g. uterine rupture, cord prolapse and abruption) should be responded to appropriately. In other situations, if the CTG abnormality persists and an instrumental vaginal delivery is not feasible, then a fetal blood sample should be performed.

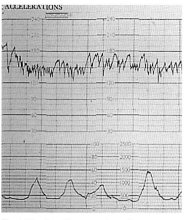

Fig 147 Reactive normal cardiotocogram.

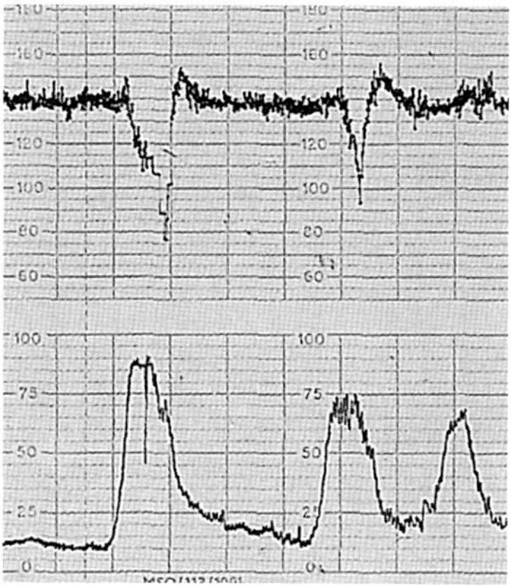

Fig 148 Early decelerations.

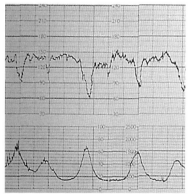

Fig 149 Variable decelerations.

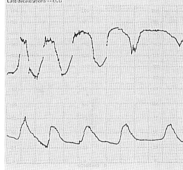

Fig 150 Late decelerations, tachycardia and reduced baseline variability.

Fetal blood sampling (FBS)

Aim
To discover whether a pathological FHR is due to fetal hypoxia. If this is confirmed, delivery can be expedited and severe asphyxia prevented.

Equipment
pH meter, a cold light source, ethyl chloride spray, antiseptic lotions and cream, silicone jelly, small magnet with iron 'fleas' to stir the sample and a prepacked tray (amnioscopes, long instruments, 2-mm guarded blade, heparinized capillary tubes and swabs) (Fig 151).

Procedure
Place the mother in the left lateral position. Clean and drape the vulva. Insert an appropriately sized amnioscope through the cervix up against the fetal scalp. Attach the light source. Clean the fetal scalp and smear it with silicone jelly. An assistant sprays the fetal scalp with ethyl chloride to produce hyperaemia. The scalp is stabbed once with the guarded blade (Fig 152). A continuous column of blood (10-30 µL), free of air bubbles, is collected in the capillary tube (Fig 153). Haemostasis is secured by pressure to the fetal scalp.

Interpretation
- pH >7.25, base excess ≤10: normal.
- pH 7.20-7.25: borderline; repeat within 30 min.
- pH <7.20 or base excess ≥10, or if a sample is not achieved due to technical problems: delivery should be expedited.

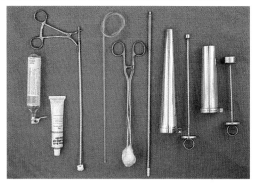

Fig 151　Fetal scalp pH instruments.

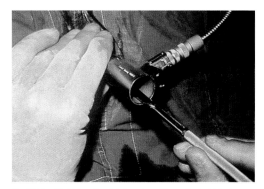

Fig 152　Stabbing the fetal scalp with protected blade.

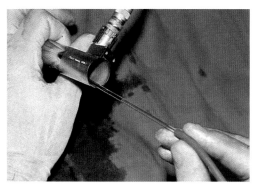

Fig 153　Aspiration of fetal blood.

Analgesia in labour

The mother should decide whether she wants pain relief in labour, although the availability may vary. Ambulation and the use of a birthing ball are encouraged. The presence of a supportive birthing partner is of proven benefit. For low-risk women, labour and even delivery can be undertaken in a warm bath (Fig 154). Psychological/relaxation methods may help. Antenatal education is an integral part of the process.

Non-pharma-cological

Aromatherapy   A newer technique practised by some midwives (Fig 155).

Transcutaneous nerve stimulation   'TENS' (Fig 156) is usually only effective in early labour and with relatively mild contractions. It is based on the 'gate control' theory of pain sensation.

Pharma-cological

Entonox®   A mixture of nitrous oxide (50%) and oxygen (50%) (Fig 157) is used by the mother, often towards the end of the first stage and during the early part of the second stage. Effective and safe for mother and baby but may cause nausea, giddiness and loss of control.

Opiates   Intramuscular pethidine (50-150 mg) with or without an antiemetic is widely used. The advantages of opiates are ease of administration, rapid effect, low incidence of serious side-effects, and antagonists are available. Patient-controlled analgesia with intravenous opiates is an alternative approach. The disadvantages include inadequate analgesia in 40%, and vomiting is common. Neonatal respiratory depression can occur if the administration to delivery interval is less than 2 h. However, the effect is reversible with naloxone.

Epidural anaesthesia

This is the most effective analgesic method, but experience in its use is essential.

Indications
On request, prolonged labour, breech presentation, multiple pregnancy, preterm labour, forceps delivery, hypertension, maternal distress/exhaustion.

Contraindications
Lack of experienced personnel, infection at insertion site, spinal abnormalities, coagulation abnormalities, hypovolaemia, acute fetal compromise.

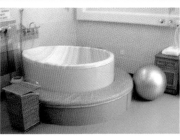

Fig 154   Birthing pool.

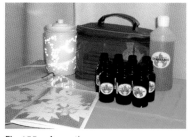

Fig 155   Aromatherapy.

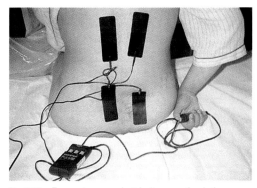

Fig 156   Transcutaneous electrical nerve stimulation (TENS).

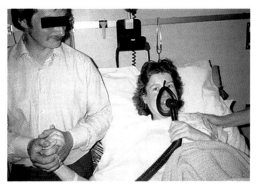

Fig 157   Entonox.

Technique

The materials used are prepacked (Fig 158). Insertion is in the left lateral or upright positions. The epidural needle is inserted through the L3/L4 or L4/L5 intervertebral disc space until there is a loss of resistance (Fig 159), indicating that the epidural (extradural) space has been reached. The cannula is then threaded through the needle into this space (Fig 160).

Externally, the cannula is strapped up over the back and shoulder for ease of access (Fig 161) with a bacterial filter attached. Bupivacaine alone (repeated injections or as an infusion for continuous analgesia) or with opiates (e.g. fentanyl) are the drugs commonly used. The dose is tailored to the patient's size and response.

Blood pressure, respiration and FHR (continuous) are carefully monitored. The aim is to 'block' (anaesthetize) T10-L1. An epidural or a single subarachnoid/intrathecal ('spinal') injection can provide regional analgesia for procedures such as manual removal of placenta or caesarean section.

Complications

- Dural puncture (headache).
- Total spinal block (loss of sensory and motor function, unconsciousness, hypotension, apnoea).
- Hypotension (due to caval compression, reduced venous return and cardiac output, and pooled blood in splanchnic bed).
- Motor paralysis.
- Urinary retention.
- Toxic reactions.
- Rarely, an aseptic meningitis.

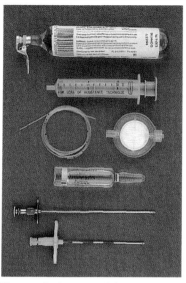

Fig 158　Equipment needed for an epidural.

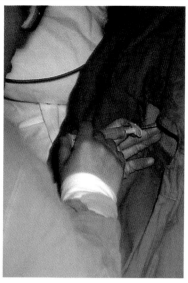

Fig 159　Epidural anaesthesia: insertion of needle.

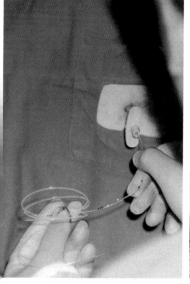

Fig 160　Epidural anaesthesia: threading the cannula through the needle.

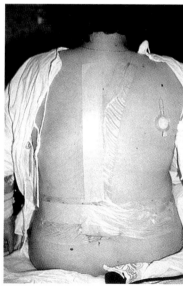

Fig 161　Epidural anaesthesia: in situ.

17 Episiotomy

The decision to perform an episiotomy requires considerable experience and judgement. Not all mothers will experience a severe perineal tear, and certainly most multiparae will be able to have a delivery with an intact perineum. The previous practice of episiotomy for all primigravidae was not evidence-based and should be discouraged.

Indications
Avoidance of inevitable severe perineal tear, to expedite delivery late in second stage when there is evidence of fetal compromise, most forceps deliveries (to avoid severe tears) and breech delivery.

Technique
The episiotomy (posterolateral) should be performed with sharp scissors at the correct time (too early results in unnecessary blood loss, while too late may end with a perineal tear anyway), with adequate local or regional (epidural or spinal block) analgesia and repaired properly as quickly as possible after delivery.

If episiotomy is necessary, then the perineum initially is infiltrated with 10 mL of 1% lidocaine (lignocaine) as it becomes distended (Fig 162).

A mediolateral direction for the episiotomy (extending posterolaterally from the fourchette) is chosen as this limits the risk of extension into the anal sphincter (Fig 163). The episiotomy should be performed during a contraction when the perineum is maximally distended.

Episiotomy repair

Technique
The patient is placed in the lithotomy position and the vulva and perineum cleaned and gowned. Lighting and the field of view should be adequate. There should be adequate analgesia using local anaesthetic or regional analgesia.

Vaginal skin The apex of the vaginal incision must be clearly identified (Fig 164). The vaginal skin is repaired with a continuous suture of polyglycolic acid, starting just above the apex of the incision (Fig 165). Care must be taken to ensure an even apposition of the vaginal skin edges. The suture is tied at the level of the hymenal remnants.

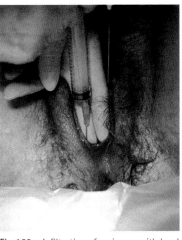

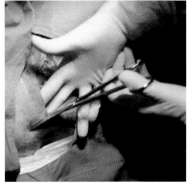

Fig 163   Cutting a right mediolateral episiotomy.

Fig 162   Infiltration of perineum with local anaesthetic.

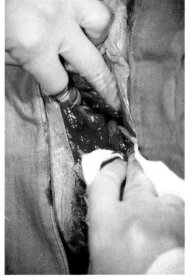

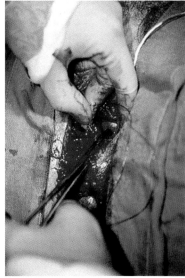

Fig 164   Inspection of apex of vaginal incision.

Fig 165   Vaginal suture.

Perineal tissues   On completion of the vaginal suturing the defect in the perineum should be approximately elliptical. The deep tissues of the perineum are repaired with interrupted sutures of polyglycolic acid. The perineal body sutures (Fig 166) are inserted with care to avoid penetration of the rectum and at right-angles to the axis of the defect.

Perineal skin   The perineal skin should be repaired with a rapidly dissolving polyglycolic acid suture. Interrupted sutures (Fig 167) or a subcuticular technique may be used. After the repair has been completed, a vaginal examination is performed (Fig 168) to check that no swabs have been left in the vagina and that there is no remaining defect or haematoma. Finally, a rectal examination is performed to confirm that no sutures have penetrated the rectal mucosa (Fig 169).

Aftercare

Adequate analgesia should be offered to the mother, both systemic (oral or per rectum analgesics) and topical (ice-packs, witch hazel/hemalis water). Complications include haemorrhage, dehiscence, infection and fistula formation.

Perineal tears

Management
First-degree (skin only) and second-degree (skin and perineal body) perineal tears are managed and repaired in the same way as an episiotomy (above).

More serious tears include the anal sphincter (third-degree) and/or rectum (fourth-degree). They are repaired usually in the operating room under general or regional anesthesia by an experienced obstetrician. The rectum and anus are first repaired with fine interrupted polyglycolic acid sutures (leaving the knots in the rectal lumen), and then the edges of the sphincter are overlapped with non-dissolvable sutures. The residual second-degree tear is then repaired in the usual manner. The mother is given a high-fibre diet, laxative/aperient and antibiotics afterwards.

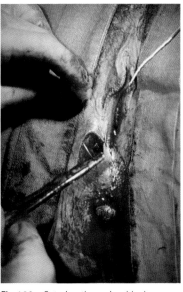

Fig 166 Suturing the perineal body.

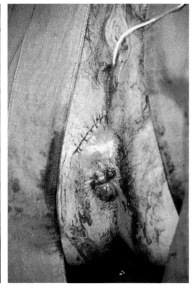

Fig 167 Sutured perineal skin.

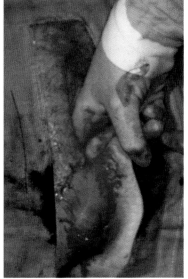

Fig 168 Vaginal examination.

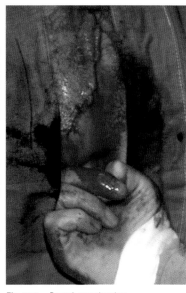

Fig 169 Rectal examination.

Indications

The decision to end a pregnancy is taken when it is considered that the infant will be safer if delivered, or the risk to the maternal health of continuing with the pregnancy outweighs the risk of delivery to the baby.

If the risk of labour is unacceptable, then delivery should be by caesarean section. In other cases, labour can be induced. Maternal indications may include hypertension, diabetes and cardiac disease. Fetal indications may include growth retardation, multiple pregnancy and premature rupture of the membranes at term.

Contraindications

- *Absolute*: include a fetal lie that is not longitudinal, poor fetal condition, an unavoidable obstruction to vaginal delivery (e.g. lower segment fibroid), a previous upper segment caesarean section ('classical') or history of uterine rupture.
- *Relative*: grand multiparity, previous lower segment uterine scar, breech presentation, prematurity (less than 34 weeks).

Methods

If the cervix is very favourable for induction, membrane rupture (amniotomy) with an amnihook (Fig 170) may be all that is required. An intravenous infusion of an oxytocic agent is often necessary after an amniotomy.

Most inductions are initiated with prostaglandin E_2 in various formulations; the majority of inductions use vaginal tablets or pessaries, or gel (Fig 171). Repeated doses may be necessary to bring the cervix to a point that will allow amniotomy and commencement of oxytocin. Vaginal delivery of a dead fetus or one with a lethal malformation can be undertaken using other methods (e.g.extra-amniotic prostaglandin E_2 administered via an endocervical catheter, or a combination of antiprogesterone and prostaglandin E_2 given orally and vaginally).

Complications

Iatrogenic prematurity, hyperstimulation (Fig 172), infection, or failed induction. Large doses of synthetic oxytocin can produce neonatal jaundice and water intoxication of mother and baby.

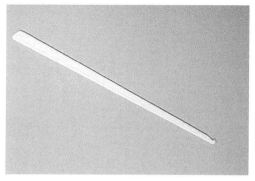

Fig 170   Amnihook.

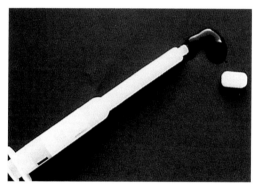

Fig 171   Gel and tablet prostaglandin formulations.

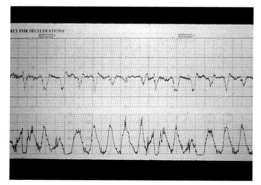

Fig 172   Uterine hyperstimulation (more than five contractions every 10 min).

19 > Forceps

Forceps

Prerequisites
- A valid indication must exist (see below).
- Suitable presentation.
- Absence of cephalopelvic disproportion or excessive moulding.
- No fetal head palpable per abdomen.
- Known position of the fetal head.
- Full dilatation of the cervix.
- Adequate analgesia.
- Empty bladder.
- Adequate uterine contractions.

Indications
- Maternal conditions in which prolonged expulsive efforts may be contraindicated (e.g. cardiac disease, hypertension, dural puncture).
- Presumed/confirmed fetal compromise in the second stage.
- Cord prolapse in the second stage.
- Poor progress in the second stage due to maternal exhaustion or occipitoposterior position.
- For delivery of the head in a breech delivery.

There is no evidence that elective forceps delivery of low-birthweight infants confers any benefits to the baby.

Types of forceps (Fig 173)
- *Non-rotational*: suitable for occipitoanterior fetal head positions. They have a cephalic curve and a pelvic curve (e.g. Neville Barnes, Wrigley's, Simpson's).
- *Rotational*: suitable for rotating transverse or occipitoposterior positions to occipitoanterior. They only have a cephalic curve (e.g. Kielland's).

Procedure (non-rotational)
Check examination findings and place the mother into the lithotomy position. Clean, gown and catheterize. Analgesia must be adequate: regional analgesia (e.g. epidural) or local anaesthetic with 1% lidocaine (lignocaine) (pudendal and perineal blocks). The forceps blades are lubricated and guided alongside the fetal head (left blade first) (Fig 174). Traction is applied with a contraction and maternal effort (Fig 175). An episiotomy is normally performed and the head delivered gently with protection of the perineum as for a normal delivery (Fig 176). The forceps blades are removed.

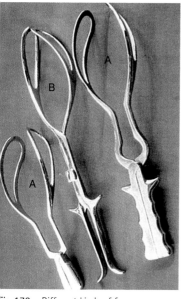

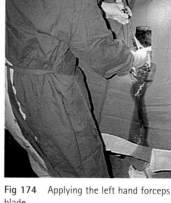

Fig 174 Applying the left hand forceps blade.

Fig 173 Different kinds of forceps.

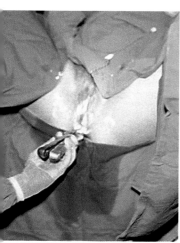

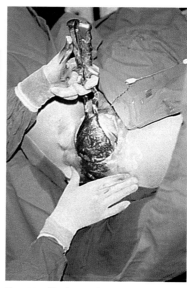

g 175 Applying traction with forceps.

Fig 176 Head crowning.

Indications
Same as for forceps, but cannot be used during a breech delivery. Use at less than full dilatation is not accepted in the USA or by many obstetricians elsewhere.

Instruments
Stainless steel or plastic cup with suction tube and sometimes a chain. Variable cup diameter (40 mm, 50 mm, or 60 mm). A suction machine is usually required, although newer ventouse cups are hand-held with a built-in suction pump. Specially designed rotational ventouse cups are available with side-fitting suction arms. These are suitable when the position is any other than occipitoanterior (Fig 177).

Technique
A suitably sized cup is applied as near to the flexion point as possible (just anterior to the posterior fontanelle) and a vacuum is created by means of a hand or electric pump (Fig 178). The pressure is initially increased to 0.2 kg/cm², then, after having checked there is no vagina or cervix included under the rim, the pressure is increased gradually to 0.8 kg/cm². There is no advantage in making this process take longer than 2 min. Traction is then applied (Fig 179), coinciding with uterine contractions and maternal pushing; the suction is released when the head passes through the introitus.

Complications
Fetal scalp abrasions and cephalohaematomas are common. Retinal haemorrhages, intracranial haemorrhage and scalp necrosis occur rarely. The ventouse should not be used if there is any risk of a fetal bleeding disorder.

Advantages
The vacuum requires less analgesia and carries less risk of maternal trauma than the forceps. It takes only marginally longer to perform than a forceps delivery.

Disadvantages
Some argue that it is relatively inefficient in cases of malrotation. Failure rates with the ventouse are higher than with forceps. It cannot be used in face presentation or in a vaginal breech delivery for delivering the aftercoming head.

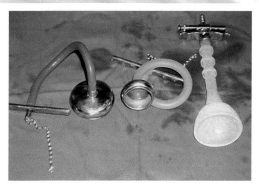

Fig 177   Different kinds of ventouse cups.

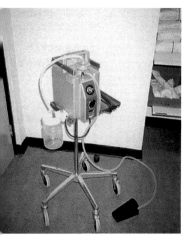

Fig 178   Suction machine.

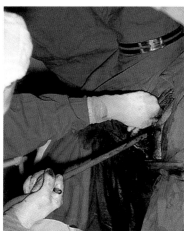

Fig 179   Applying traction with a ventouse.

Incidence

Varies with policies and populations at different centres: currently, 20% in the UK and 20-25% in North America. May be elective (planned in advance) or an emergency. Maternal and perinatal mortality and morbidity are higher when the operation is an emergency.

Indications

Routine/elective caesarean section (CS)
- Previous CS with recurrent cause (e.g. true cephalopelvic disproportion).
- Two or more previous CS.
- Breech presentation.
- Placenta praevia.
- Unstable lie.
- Maternal disease (e.g. severe cardiac disease, untreated berry aneurysm, recent retinal detachment).
- Maternal choice (highly controversial).
- Twins when the first twin is anything other than a vertex presentation, and higher-order multiple gestations.

Emergency CS
- Presumed/confirmed fetal compromise ('fetal distress'): i.e. abnormal cardiotocography, acidosis on fetal blood sampling, cord prolapse or abruption before or during the first stage of labour.
- Obstructed labour (e.g. pelvic cyst/fibroid).
- Prolonged labour due to dysfunctional uterine activity, malposition or true cephalopelvic disproportion.
- Bleeding from placenta praevia.
- Delivery for maternal risk (e.g. uncontrollable hypertension, eclampsia) where prompt vaginal delivery is not feasible (usually preterm).
- Contractions/labour in a pregnancy with a date for elective CS for any of the reasons listed above.

Technique

Following induction of general or regional (spinal) anaesthesia, the patient is catheterized, the abdomen is cleaned with antiseptic (Fig 180) and draped with sterile towels. The abdomen is opened with either a lower transverse incision (Fig 181) or a midline subumbilical incision.

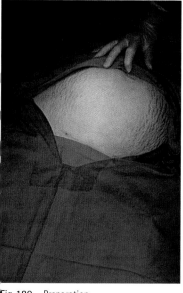

Fig 180   Preparation.

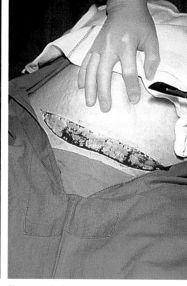

Fig 181   Incision.

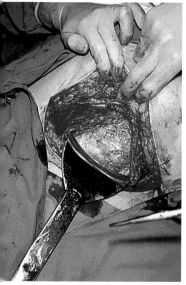

Fig 182   Exposure of the lower uterine segment.

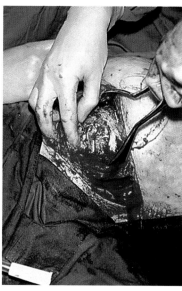

Fig 183   Delivery of the head with forceps.

Types of operation

Lower segment   This is the most common approach, used in 99% of cases. The uterovesical peritoneum is reflected (Fig 182) and the lower segment opened with a transverse incision. The risk of rupture in subsequent labour is low (about 0.3%).

Upper segment   This approach was used for several centuries, hence its description as 'classical'. A vertical incision is made in the upper segment of the uterus. It is associated with a greater blood loss, higher risk of rupture in a subsequent labour (4-9%) and greater risk of bowel adhesions and postoperative ileus.

Indications for classical CS are:

- Transverse lie which cannot readily be converted to longitudinal (e.g. prolapsed arm).
- Certain uterine abnormalities (e.g. fibroids in the lower segment).
- Some cases of placenta praevia.
- For delivery of some low-birthweight babies (particularly with oligohydramnios). A poorly formed lower segment may make delivery difficult and traumatic through a transverse incision.
- Dense adhesions obscuring the lower segment.

Procedure

The head is delivered either manually or with forceps (Figs 183, 184). An oxytocic agent is administered intravenously to the mother and the placenta is delivered by cord traction (Fig 185). The uterus is repaired in two layers of continuous absorbable sutures (Fig 186). The abdomen is closed in layers (Fig 187). There are variations in the technique of closure of both uterus and abdomen. Postoperative attention is paid to analgesia, physiotherapy, mobilization and assistance with feeding.

Complications

These include haemorrhage, infection (e.g. wound, urinary), thromboembolic disease, visceral damage, paralytic ileus, infertility and increased risk of CS and placenta praevia in a future pregnancy.

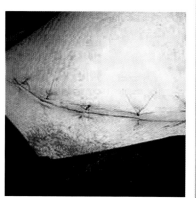

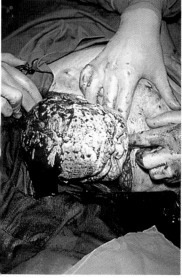

Fig 184   Head delivered.

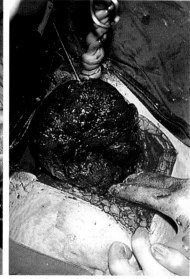

Fig 185   Delivery of the placenta.

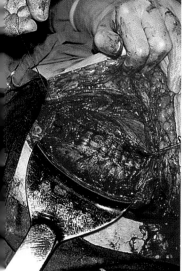

Fig 186   Uterine repair.

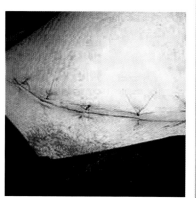

Fig 187   Skin sutures.

Incidence

The incidence of spontaneous (naturally occurring) twins is about 1 in 80 pregnancies. Spontaneous higher-order multiples are much less common: triplets 1 in 8000, quadruplets 1 in 80 000. Assisted reproductive techniques (e.g. use of clomifene and in vitro fertilization) have increased the numbers of multiple gestations above these estimates.

Types

Monochorionic (MC, identical)   Result from fertilization of single ovum that divides into two embryos. Rarely share the same sac (monoamniotic, 1%) and very rarely are conjoined (Fig 188). No racial or familial predisposition. Characterized on ultrasound at the end of the first trimester by a thin dividing membrane which joins the uterine wall as a 'T'-shaped insertion (Fig 189).

Dichorionic (DC, non-identical/fraternal)   Result from multiple ovulation and fertilization. Strong familial and racial (e.g. Nigerian) predisposition. More frequent with greater maternal age, parity, height and obesity. The MC/DC ratio is 1:4. Characterized on ultrasound at the end of the first trimester by a thick dividing membrane that joins the uterine wall as a 'V' or 'lambda' sign (Fig 190).

Diagnosis

Usually detected now at the dating or routine detailed ultrasound. May also present as 'large-for-dates', hyperemesis, a raised serum α-fetoprotein, or early hypertension/pre-eclampsia. Clinical diagnosis is made by palpating more than two poles or detecting two fetal hearts.

General complications

With the exception of postmaturity, every complication of pregnancy is increased, including preterm labour, pre-eclampsia and fetal growth restriction, accounting for about 10% of perinatal deaths. Monochorionic twins have a much higher perinatal mortality as they run the risk of twin–twin transfusion syndrome.

Specific complications

Twin–twin transfusion syndrome   Complicates only monochorionic twin pregnancies. A mismatch in

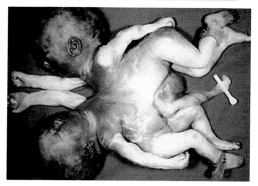

Fig 188   Conjoined twins.

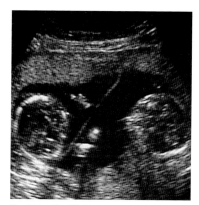

Fig 189   The 'T' sign of monochorionic twins.

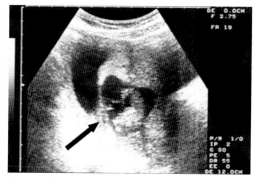

Fig 190   The lambda sign of dichorionic twins.

arteriovenous connections across the shared placenta causes an unequal distribution of blood. The 'donor' twin is anaemic and growth-restricted, with oligohydramnios. The 'recipient' twin becomes plethoric/polycythaemic and large-for-dates, with polyhydramnios. The effect is obvious at delivery (Fig 191). Untreated, the preterm delivery and perinatal mortality rates are extremely high. The problem can be corrected by laser treatment to the placenta.

Monoamniotic twins   Comprise 1% of cases. Can result in cord entanglement (Fig 192) and twin entrapment at delivery.

Antenatal care
In addition to routine antenatal care:

- Dietary supplementation of iron and folate.
- More frequent antenatal checks.
- Detailed scan at 20 weeks (higher rate of fetal anomalies) (Fig 193).
- Monthly growth scans thereafter (more often if discordant).
- Vigilance for preterm labour (approximately 10% deliver at less than 28 weeks; 30% deliver at less than 37 weeks).

Many advocate increased surveillance of monochorionic twins (from 18 weeks). Induction of labour at 38-40 weeks is often advised if spontaneous delivery has not occurred.

Mode of delivery
Most obstetricians would advise a vaginal delivery with a vertex/vertex presentation. A caesarean section is recommended if the first twin is any other presentation than cephalic or if either twin is compromised.

Labour and delivery
Continuously monitor both fetuses. Epidural block is the preferred mode of analgesia. Delivery of the first twin is as for a singleton. Delay in delivery of the second twin carries an increased risk of asphyxia. An oxytocin infusion should be ready (contractions tend to subside after delivery of the first baby). The abdomen is palpated to determine the lie and presentation of the second twin. A transverse lie is converted to longitudinal either by external version or by grasping a foot vaginally. With the next contraction, the mother recommences pushing and the membranes are ruptured. Delivery of the second twin may be spontaneous or assisted. Two paediatricians and double resuscitation facilities should be available at delivery. There is an increased risk of primary postpartum haemorrhage.

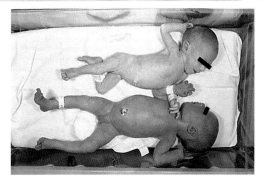

Fig 191   Twin–twin transfusion syndrome.

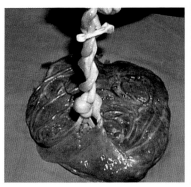

Fig 192   Cord entanglement of monoamniotic twins.

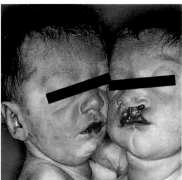

Fig 193   Risk of congenital anomaly.

Incidence

Falls with advancing gestation: 25% at 30 weeks, 3% at 40 weeks.

Aetiology

- Uterine anomalies (e.g. fibroids, bicornate uterus).
- Fetal anomalies (e.g. hydrocephalus, anencephaly).
- Multiple pregnancy.
- Placenta praevia.

  In most cases, no cause is identified.

Management

Confirm with ultrasound from 36 weeks and exclude obvious causes (see above). Options include:

- *External cephalic version*: this approach should be encouraged in otherwise uncomplicated pregnancies. The fetus is manipulated through the anterior abdominal and uterine walls into a cephalic presentation, aided by tocolysis. 40-60% success rates.
- *Elective caesarean section (CS)*: should be advised if external cephalic version fails, as the evidence suggests this carries least fetal risk.
- *Vaginal breech delivery*: has higher perinatal morbidity/ mortality rates (especially if macrosomia, primiparity or a footling presentation). Early recourse to emergency CS if poor progress or fetal compromise.

Vaginal breech delivery

Continuous fetal heart rate monitoring should be instigated. Slow progress and abnormal cardiotocogram are commonly managed by CS, even in the second stage. Fetal buttock sampling for pH and use of oxytocin are controversial. An epidural prevents premature pushing and allows manipulation. Pushing is encouraged once the buttocks/feet (Fig 194) are visible, and a generous episiotomy is made with their delivery. Delivery to the umbilicus is by maternal effort alone. If the legs are extended, their delivery is assisted by abduction and flexion at the knees (Fig 195). The arms usually lie across the chest, and maternal effort is sufficient to deliver the shoulders. A finger in the antecubital fossa can be used to bring down extended arms (Fig 196). The fetus is either allowed to hang or delivered along the attendant's arm until the hairline is visible. Delivery of the head is controlled by the Mauriceau–Smellie–Veit manoeuvre or by applying forceps after an assistant has lifted the feet (Fig 197).

Complications

These are discussed in Chapter 24.

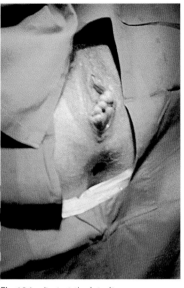

Fig 194   Feet at the introitus.

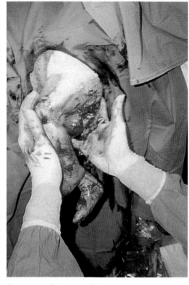

Fig 195   Delivery of the legs.

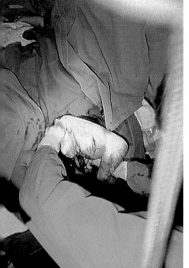

Fig 196   Delivery of the arms.

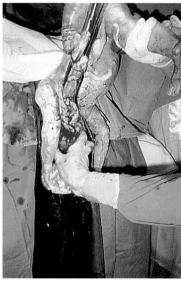

Fig 197   Delivery of the head with the aid of forceps.

Cephalohaematoma

Definition
Fluctuant mass loosely attached under the periosteum of cranial bones (commonly parietal) and not crossing the suture lines (Fig 198). May contribute to anaemia and jaundice but usually resolves over several weeks.

Incidence
0.5-2.5% of vaginal deliveries.

Aetiology
May follow spontaneous delivery but more commonly follows forceps or ventouse (3%).

Facial nerve palsy

Presents as asymmetry of the face on crying (Fig 199). Most cases resolve within days.

Incidence
Approximately 0.25% of births

Aetiology
Compression of the facial nerve distal to the stylomastoid foramen during labour or delivery. More common with forceps, but can follow normal delivery due to pressure on a maternal bony prominence or the fetal shoulder.

Management
Protect the eye which cannot be closed (lower motor neuron lesion).

Injuries confined to instrumental delivery

Ventouse

Scalp ecchymoses and artificial caput (the chignon) always occur with ventouse delivery. Scalp abrasions (8%) are more likely with metal cups and if the application time is prolonged (maximum duration should be 15 min) (Fig 200); they take longer to heal and necrosis can occur. Aspiration of cerebral tissue through open fontanelles has also been reported.

Forceps

Facial pressure marks are common (Fig 201), abrasions less so. Skull fracture is a rare but very serious complication.

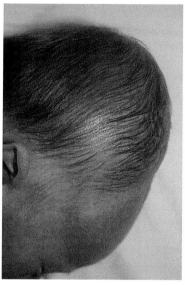

Fig 198 Cephalohaematoma.

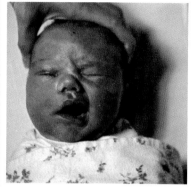

Fig 199 Facial nerve palsy.

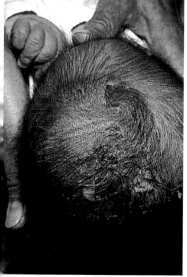

Fig 200 Ventouse abrasion.

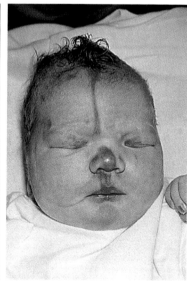

Fig 201 Forceps mark.

Injuries associated with vaginal breech delivery

Vaginal breech delivery predisposes to certain types of injury, including bruising to genitalia, spinal cord lesions, peripheral nerve palsies, fractured bones and intracranial bleeding. Injuries to the liver (Fig 202) or spleen can be avoided by minimizing handling of the breech.

Brachial plexus injuries

Types

Erb's palsy   Incidence 97%. Stretching, bruising or avulsion of C5 and C6 nerve roots causes internal rotation of the arm with extension and adduction of the hand (Fig 90). Rarely, a phrenic nerve palsy also occurs.

Klumpke's palsy   Incidence 3%. Lesion of C8 and T1. Weakness of hand. Rarely with Horner syndrome.

Aetiology
Traction on brachial plexus during delivery. More common after shoulder dystocia and vaginal breech delivery.

Prognosis
80% recover completely in 3-6 months. Occasionally there is severe permanent deficit, resulting in a functionless short limb.

Tentorial tear

Aetiology
Hypoxia renders the brain oedematous and its supporting membranes rigid and prone to damage (Fig 203). Excessive moulding, prematurity, breech and instrumental delivery are further predisposing factors.

Clinical features
The infant is usually flaccid, pale and difficult to resuscitate at birth. Survivors have a high incidence of neurological sequelae.

Other injuries

Subconjunctival haemorrhages, avulsion or infection at the site of fetal scalp electrodes (Fig 204) and lacerations at the time of caesarean section (Fig 205) many of which are avoidable.

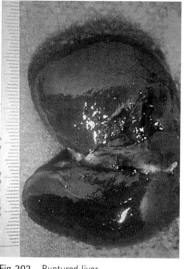

Fig 202   Ruptured liver.

Fig 203   Tentorial tear.

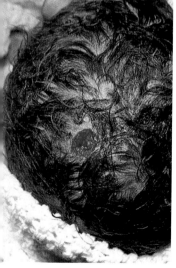

Fig 204   Avulsion of scalp skin by fetal
scalp electrode.

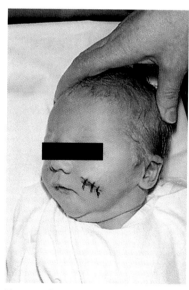

Fig 205   Facial laceration at caesarean
section.

Definition

The interval taken to return to the normal non-pregnant state following delivery. Definitions vary in different countries. For many it is taken as 6 weeks, although most anatomical changes are complete within 2 weeks. In the UK, it is a statutory requirement for mothers to be seen daily for 10-14 days by a midwife who routinely checks blood pressure, temperature, scars, lochia, breasts and involution of the uterus (Fig 206). The midwife also checks that the infant is well and advises on feeding difficulties.

Complications

Puerperal sepsis   Defined as a temperature of 38°C or more within 14 days of delivery. The usual causes include:

- Breast infection.
- Urinary infection.
- Wound infection (following caesarean section).
- Thrombophlebitis (legs or drip sites).
- Thromboembolic disease.
- Pelvic infection (with or without retained placental tissue).

Perineal complications   Perineal pain is extremely common following vaginal delivery and results from bruising (Fig 207), oedema (Fig 208) and infection. Analgesia, frequent bathing and removal of any tight sutures provide symptomatic relief.

Vaginal complications   Vaginal haematomas (Fig 209) are less common. Presentation is with increasingly severe vaginal/rectal pain, usually within 6 h of delivery. The pain is often refractory to opiate analgesia, and the haematoma is palpable on vaginal or rectal examination. Management is by surgical evacuation of the clot, haemostasis and resuturing of the vagina and perineum. The amount of blood contained may be sufficient to make the patient anaemic. Small haematomas can be treated conservatively.

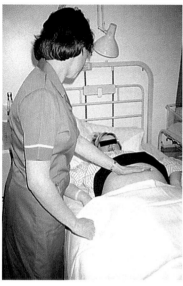

Fig 206   A postnatal check.

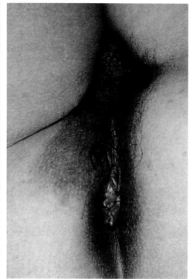

Fig 207   Perineal bruising.

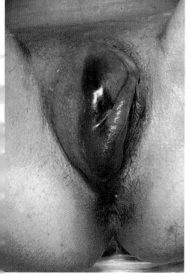

Fig 208   Perineal oedema.

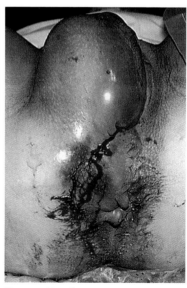

Fig 209   Vulval/vaginal haematoma.

Other complications

- Haemorrhoids are prone to thrombosis and prolapse at delivery, resulting in pain and irritation (Fig 210).
- Subconjunctival haemorrhages (Fig 211) may result from maternal expulsive efforts during the second stage. They are asymptomatic and resolve spontaneously.
- Wound infection or haematoma (Fig 212) follow 10% of caesarean sections. They delay healing and, when associated with a vertical incision, occasionally give rise to wound dehiscence (rare with a transverse incision). Chest infection, thromboembolism, ileus, urinary tract infection and anaemia are also more common than following vaginal delivery.
- Uterine infection (endometritis) is usually at the placental site and presents with pyrexia, abdominal discomfort and vaginal bleeding. Treatment is with antibiotics and analgesia.
- Deep venous thrombosis and pulmonary embolus are more common following caesarean section. Pulmonary embolus is a leading cause of maternal mortality.

Complications of breastfeeding

Engorgement of the breasts normally occurs on days 2-4. Mastitis (Fig 213) is relatively common and starts with reddening and tenderness, progressing to an oedematous induration with fever and malaise.

Aetiology
Staphylococci or streptococci, often from the baby during suckling, particularly with a cracked nipple and associated stasis of milk in breast lobule or blocked duct.

Management
Antibiotics (flucloxacillin), analgesia and regular breast-emptying (infection is not a contraindication to continuing breastfeeding in a healthy baby). Neglected mastitis can progress to abscess formation requiring surgical drainage or aspiration.

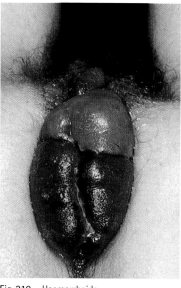

Fig 210   Haemorrhoids.

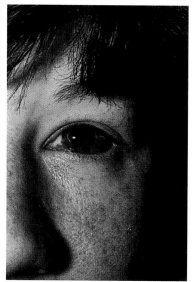

Fig 211   Subconjunctival haemorrhages.

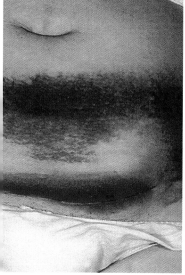

Fig 212   Wound haematoma and bruising.

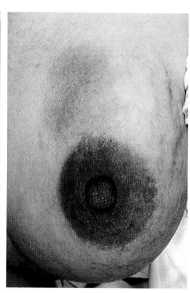

Fig 213   Mastitis.

Following pregnancy, sexual activity may be resumed as soon as it is comfortable to do so. This may take several weeks if a woman has had a perineal repair. Most anatomical changes of pregnancy have regressed by 2-4 weeks. Endocrine changes take longer; return to fertility is variable and may be delayed for months by lactation. Non-lactating women may ovulate within 4 weeks of delivery, and return of menstruation occurs, on average, at 58 days. It is extremely rare for fully breastfeeding women to ovulate or menstruate. However, breastfeeding alone is not a recommended contraceptive method.

Hormonal methods

Some typical examples are shown in Fig 214. The combined oral contraceptive pill (COCP) should be avoided in breastfeeding women as the oestrogen content may suppress lactation. Non-lactating women may commence the COCP no sooner than 3 weeks postpartum due to the natural increase in thrombotic risk during the puerperium. The usual contraindications to the use of the COCP must also be considered (e.g. history of prior thromboembolism, cerebrovascular accident, liver disease).

Progestogen-based preparations (e.g. progestogen-only pill, progestogenic implants) do not interfere with lactation and can be started immediately. They may, however, cause erratic bleeding initially and this can be confusing and an annoyance in the postpartum period.

Intrauterine contraceptive devices

Insertion can be undertaken at any time in the puerperium (Figs 215, 216). In general, however, expulsion rates are higher when insertion is earlier and thus this is usually deferred until 6 weeks. The progestogen-based intrauterine system (Mirena) has a very low failure rate (comparable with the COCP), but can cause irregular bleeding for 3-6 months postinsertion. More traditional copper-based coils can cause menorrhagia and dysmenorrhoea and are associated with a higher risk of pelvic infection. Failure of the device increases the chances of an ectopic pregnancy or preterm miscarriage/labour.

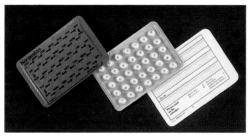

Fig 214   Various contraceptive pills.

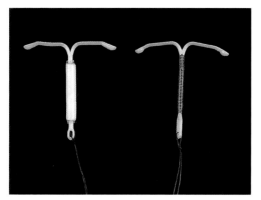

Fig 215   Intrauterine contraceptive devices.

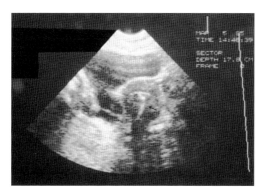

Fig 216   Ultrasound image showing an intrauterine contraceptive device.

Barrier methods

The sheath (Fig 217) is commonly used as a short-term contraceptive in the puerperium (e.g. until breastfeeding ceases and the combined pill can be prescribed, or until an intrauterine contraceptive device can be inserted at 6 weeks, or until an interval sterilization is performed). Women who have used a diaphragm (Fig 218) before pregnancy may need a different size after childbirth; this can be reassessed after 6 weeks.

Sterilization

Female

Tubal occlusion for those women wanting permanent contraception can be performed at caesarean section, although a higher failure rate is quoted (1 in 200) than for sterilizations performed at a time distant to pregnancy (1 in 300). This is probably because of the greater thickness and vascularity of the tubes.

Female sterilization is more usually performed laparoscopically. The failure rate is quoted as 1 in 300. Clips or rings are used to occlude the fallopian tubes (Fig 219). For those women conceiving after sterilization, the risk of ectopic pregnancy is substantially increased.

Sterilization should be considered an irreversible procedure. Only 40-60% of sterilization reversals are followed by an intrauterine pregnancy. Visceral (e.g. bowel) damage during laparoscopic sterilization occurs in 1 in 1000 cases and is a life-threatening complication.

Male

Male sterilization has many advantages over female procedures. The failure rate is 10 times lower, no general anaesthetic is required and the surgical complications are less serious. It does not, of course, provide the woman with control over *her* fertility.

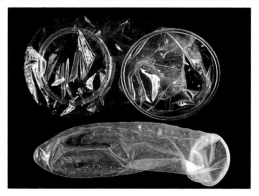

Fig 217   Male and female condoms.

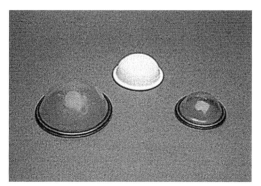

Fig 218   Contraceptive diaphragms and caps.

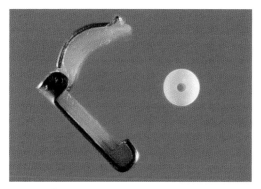

Fig 219   Sterilization clips and rings.

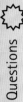

? Questions

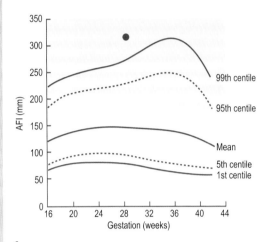

1. This amniotic fluid index (AFI) chart shows the liquor volume of a pregnancy at 28 weeks' gestation.

a. What is the diagnosis?
b. Name four causes of this.
c. Name two symptoms and two signs associated with this diagnosis.

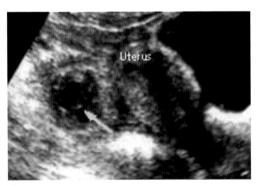

2. This is an ultrasound scan of a woman with 7 weeks of amenorrhoea, minor vaginal bleeding and a serum hCG of 3500 IU/L.

a. What is the diagnosis?
b. Name four risk factors for this condition.
c. Give three treatment options.

3. These are curettings removed from the uterus of a woman presenting at 8 weeks' amenorrhoea with vaginal bleeding and a serum hCG of 80 000 IU/L.

a. What is the diagnosis?
b. What might have been found on the ultrasound scan?
c. How would she be managed from this point onwards?

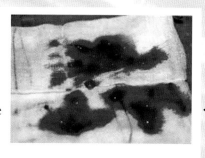

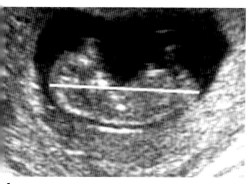

4. This is an ultrasound scan of an 11-week fetus.

a. What is this fetal biometric measurement called?
b. What is the error (i.e.±2 standard deviations) of the prediction of gestational age made using this measurement?
c. What two measurements can be used at 16 weeks' gestation to date a pregnancy?

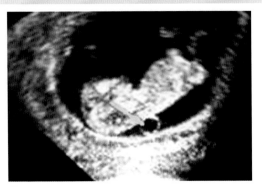

5. This ultrasound picture shows a fetus at 10 weeks' gestation.

a. What normal structure is the yellow arrow pointing to?
b. When does this first become visible and when does it disappear?
c. What is the function of this structure?

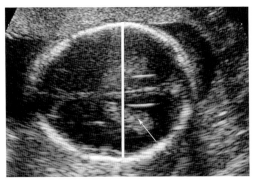

6. This ultrasound picture shows a cross-section through the fetal head at 20 weeks' gestation.

a. What measurement is shown by the white line?
b. What intracranial structure is indicated by the arrow?
c. What function does this structure have?

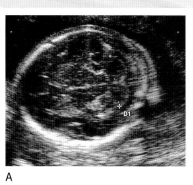 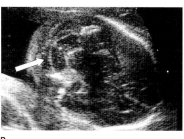

A   B

7. The calipers in image A and the arrow in image B are identifying the same structure within the fetal brain.

a. What structure is this?
b. Which of the two images is normal?
c. What condition might the fetus with the abnormal image have?

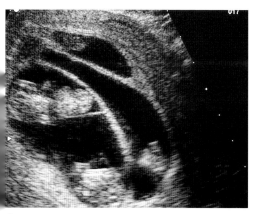

8. This ultrasound picture was taken at approximately 9 weeks' gestation.

a. What does this ultrasound picture show?
b. How might this condition have been caused?
c. Name six complications more likely in this pregnancy?

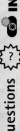
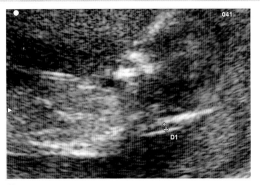

9. This ultrasound image was taken at 12 weeks' gestation.

a. What is the name of the area being measured?
b. What is the main indication for taking this measurement?
c. What alternative tests might be offered and when?

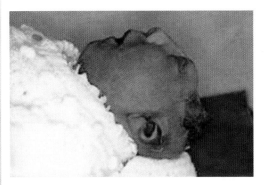

10. This baby was born to a woman who declined all forms of antenatal screening and presented at 33 weeks with a symphysiofundal height of 39 cm.

a. What abnormality is shown here?
b. How might it have been detected antenatally?
c. What caused her to have a large-for-dates uterus?

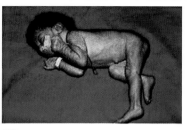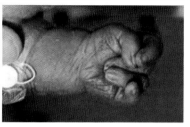

11. This baby was born with growth restriction, joint contractures and overlapping fingers with clenched fists. Antenatal scans had shown bilateral choroids plexus cysts at 20 weeks' gestation.

a. What is the diagnosis?
b. What would the karyotype be?
c. Name three other abnormalities associated with this condition.

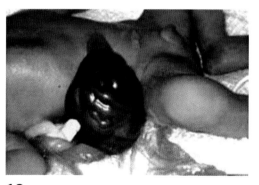

12. This baby was born at term to a couple who had declined detailed ultrasound scanning at 20 weeks' gestation.

a. What is the diagnosis?
b. If this had been detected antenatally by ultrasound what diagnostic test might have been offered?
c. What syndromes and conditions are associated with this anomaly?

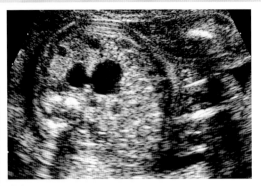

13. This ultrasound image, taken at 21 weeks' gestation, shows a cross-section through the fetal abdomen.

a. What is the name of the abnormal ultrasound feature shown here?
b. What structural abnormality causes this to occur?
c. With which syndrome is it commonly associated?

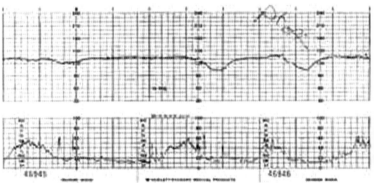

14. This cardiotocogram (CTG) is taken from a woman in labour at 38 weeks' gestation, at 2 cm dilatation. The baseline rate is 140 beats/min.

a. Name the three abnormal features shown here.
b. How would you describe this CTG?
c. What might you expect to find if you artificially ruptured the membranes?

15. This young girl is of short stature.

a. What is the diagnosis?
b. Name four other characteristic features.
c. What would be the most common antenatal ultrasound finding?

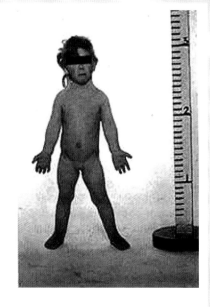

16. This baby is only a few hours old.

a. What problem is illustrated here?
b. What was the most likely method of delivery?
c. In most cases, is this permanent?

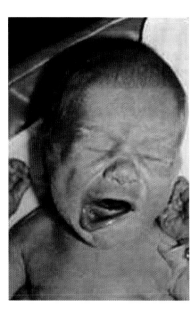

17. This term baby was born hypoxic and acidotic and subsequently developed seizures in the neonatal period.

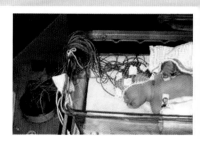

a. What is the clinical syndrome called?
b. What investigation is being performed?
c. What is the prognosis if the baby suffers seizures?

18. This infant developed a distended abdomen a few days after it was delivered prematurely for worsening maternal pre-eclampsia.

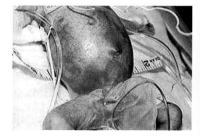

a. What is the diagnosis?
b. Which antenatal treatment can reduce the incidence of this condition?
c. How would you manage this conservatively?

19. This newborn infant has recently been delivered by elective caesarean section.

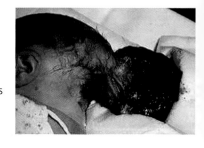

a. What congenital abnormality is present?
b. To which group of defects does this belong?
c. Which two imaging techniques would be useful in assessing this structure during pregnancy?

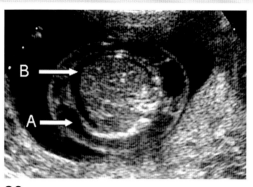

20. This ultrasound image was taken at 22 weeks' gestation and shows a cross-section through the fetal abdomen.

a. What is the diagnosis?
b. What abnormalities are indicated by the arrows A and B?
c. Name five causes.

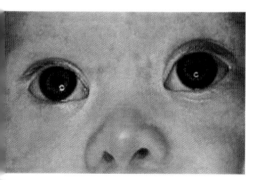

21. This baby was found to be hypotonic in the newborn period. Close examination revealed subtle dysmorphic features.

a. Name three abnormal facial features shown here.
b. What is the likely diagnosis?
c. What is the recurrence risk for this condition in a future pregnancy?

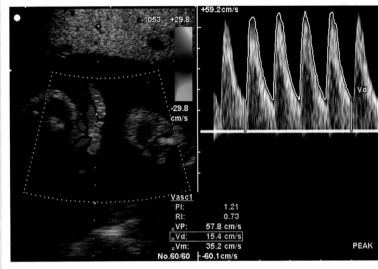

Vasc1	
PI:	1.21
RI:	0.73
_VP:	57.8 cm/s
_Vd:	15.4 cm/s
_Vm:	35.2 cm/s
No.60/60	

22. A woman at 31 weeks' gestation is admitted with pre-eclampsia for observation and fetal surveillance.

a. Which antenatal investigation is being performed here?
b. What does the waveform pattern show?
c. Why might this be abnormal in pre-eclampsia?

23. This baby was born weighing 4.5 kg following a difficult delivery.

a. What birth injury is shown in this image?
b. What is the underlying nature and mechanism of the injury?
c. Apart from fetal size, what other risk factor is associated with this condition?

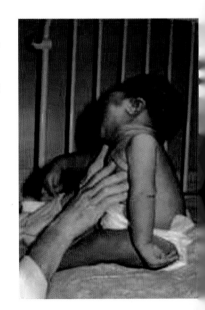

24. This woman presents at 14 weeks' gestation with a widespread vesicular rash.

a. What is the diagnosis?
b. What is the risk to the fetus at this stage of pregnancy?
c. What is the main maternal risk?

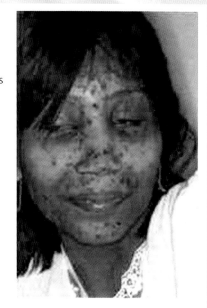

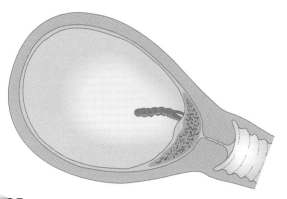

25. This line drawing shows an abnormal placental implantation.

a. What is the diagnosis and grade?
b. Name two ways in which this can present.
c. Name three risk factors for this problem.

26. This stillborn infant was found to have a malformed nose and abnormal ears.

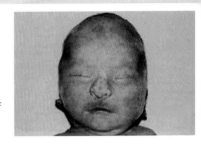

a. What name is given to this pattern of facial dysmorphism?
b. What causes this appearance?
c. What was found on examination of the lungs at postmortem?

27. This image was taken at the time of laparoscopy.

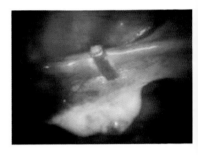

a. What procedure has been performed?
b. Name two complications of this procedure.
c. What is the failure rate of this procedure if it is performed at caesarean section?

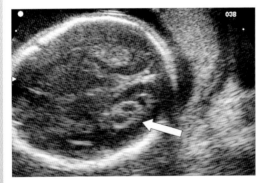

28. This ultrasound scan shows a cross-section through the fetal head at 20 weeks' gestation.

a. What abnormalities are shown by the arrow?
b. Which chromosomal abnormalities are most commonly found in association with these?
c. How common are they in normal pregnancies?

29. This newborn baby has suffered a significant birth injury.

a. How was this baby delivered?
b. What was the position of the fetal head during second stage?
c. Name three other injuries that can occur with this mode of delivery.

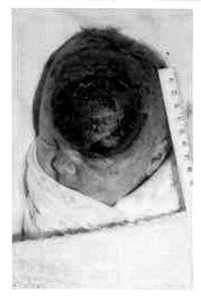

30. This newborn baby weighed 4.6 kg at 39 weeks' gestation.

a. What term is used to describe this appearance?
b. What underlying maternal condition has caused this to occur?
c. Name three neonatal complications that are more likely.

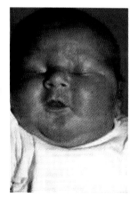

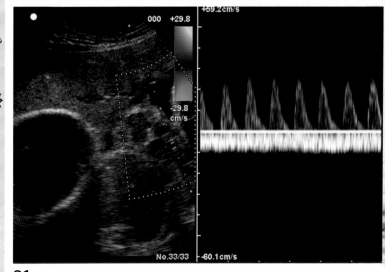

31. This umbilical artery Doppler recording was performed on a growth-restricted fetus at 35 weeks' gestation.

a. What does it show?
b. What is the likely cause of this?
c. How would you manage this case?

32. This newborn infant is 4 days old.

a. What is the term given to this appearance?
b. Name two sexually transmitted diseases that can cause it.
c. Name two management strategies for the baby and two for the mother.

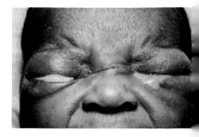

33. This congenital abnormality was noted immediately after delivery.

a. What is it called?
b. Name two conditions that might also be found in the baby.
c. What is the initial management?

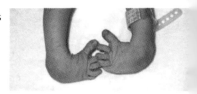

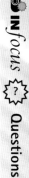

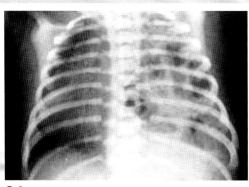

34. This neonatal chest X-ray was performed on a term baby with respiratory distress immediately after delivery. The heart was found to be shifted to the right and ventilation proved to be very difficult.

a. What is the diagnosis?
b. What are the characteristic ultrasound findings during pregnancy?
c. If this is an isolated lesion, what proportion of these babies will survive?

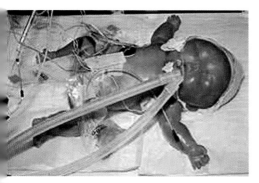

35. This newborn infant is oedematous and has cardiac failure, ascites and pulmonary oedema.

a. What is this appearance called?
b. What was the most common cause 50 years ago?
c. Name four other causes.

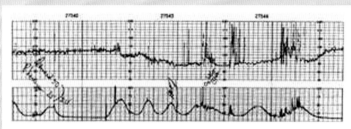

36. This cardiotocogram (CTG) is taken from a woman in labour receiving oxytocin. The baseline heart rate has been 140 beats/min during the day.

a. What abnormality is seen on this CTG?
b. What is the most likely cause?
c. What three first-aid measures would you perform?

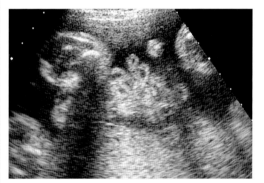

37. This image was taken at the time of a 20-week routine detailed ultrasound scan. It shows loops of bowel floating free in the amniotic cavity.

a. What is the diagnosis?
b. What is the main differential diagnosis?
c. Name the two features that distinguish these two conditions.

38. This is an image of a newborn abdomen.

a. What is this appearance called?
b. What condition most commonly gives rise to this appearance?
c. What is the most important consequence?

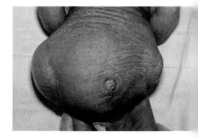

39. This newborn infant was born with partially amputated toes.

a. What is the most likely cause for this abnormality?

b. Name three other congenital defects that can be caused by the same process.

c. What is the recurrence risk for a future pregnancy?

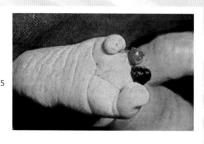

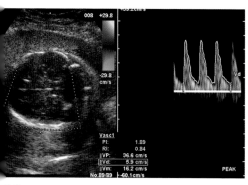

40. This image shows an antenatal Doppler waveform study.

a. Which fetal blood vessel is being studied?

b. What happens to the resistance to blood flow in a severely growth-restricted fetus?

c. What happens to the blood flow in this vessel in anaemic fetuses?

41. This pair of twins was born at 36 weeks' gestation.

a. How would you describe their growth?

b. Name two conditions that could lead to this appearance.

c. Name four complications the smaller twin might experience after birth.

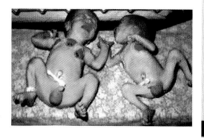

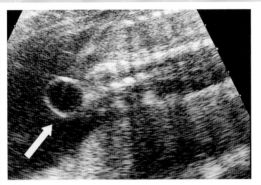

42. This ultrasound image was taken at 20 weeks' gestation.

a. What abnormality is the white arrow pointing to?
b. Name two other features that can be found in association with this defect.
c. What is the recurrence risk in a future pregnancy without any preventative treatment?

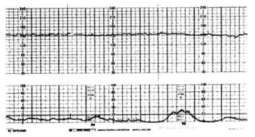

43. This cardiotocogram (CTG) is taken from a woman at 39 weeks' gestation who complained of reduced fetal movements for 3 days prior to admission and mild tightenings. The baseline is 140 beats/min and the CTG continued like this for another hour before action was taken.

a. How would you describe this CTG?
b. How would you manage the case?
c. What would you expect to find on blood gas evaluation of the umbilical artery and vein?

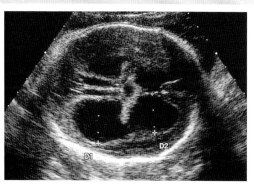

44. This scan was performed routinely at 21 weeks' gestation.

a. What structures are the calipers measuring?
b. What is this appearance called?
c. Name three causes.

45. This ultrasound picture shows a coronal section through a newborn forebrain.

a. What abnormality is visible on this scan?
b. Name two pregnancy complications that can lead to this.
c. Name two consequences for the baby.

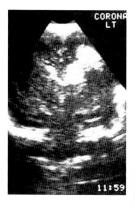

46. This baby was born vaginally following a prolonged second stage of labour due to maternal exhaustion.

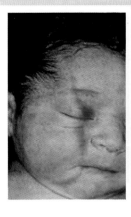

a. How was this baby delivered?
b. Name two other indications for this procedure.
c. What three complications can result from this mode of delivery?

47. This spread of chromosomes in metaphase was taken from a single cell at chorionic villus sampling.

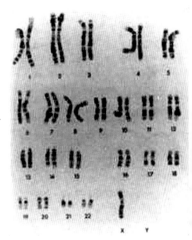

a. How would you report the fetal karyotype?
b. What name is given to this chromosomal abnormality?
c. Name five features of this condition.

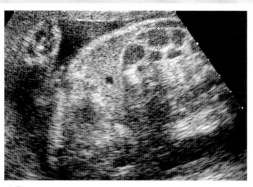

48. This ultrasound image shows a fetal kidney in longitudinal view.

a. How would you describe this kidney?

b. What two features on scan would reassure you that the fetus is producing urine?

c. What would be the most likely diagnosis if the contralateral kidney appears normal?

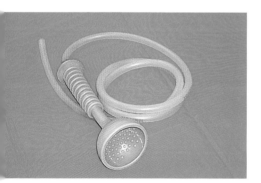

49. This instrument is commonly found on the labour ward.

a. What is this instrument?

b. Can it be used for failure to progress in second stage due to a persistent occipitoposterior position? Justify your answer.

c. Which medical conditions in the fetus contraindicate its use?

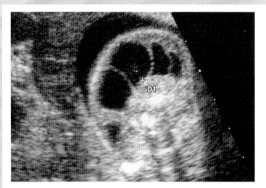

50. This ultrasound image shows a cross-section through the fetal neck at 16 weeks' gestation.

a. What abnormality is shown here?
b. Name one condition that can give rise to this appearance.
c. Which additional investigation would you offer?

51. This newborn baby has a widespread vesicular rash.

a. Which two common viral infections transmitted from the mother may be responsible?
b. Name four consequences to the newborn of infection with these viruses.
c. Which drug is used to treat neonates with these infections?

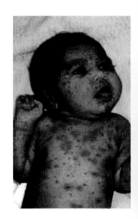

52. This abdominal X-ray was taken from a 4-day-old baby born at 28 weeks' gestation.

a. What is the likely diagnosis?
b. Name three other complications of prematurity.
c. How can the incidence of these complications be reduced?

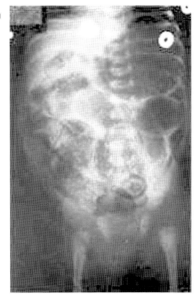

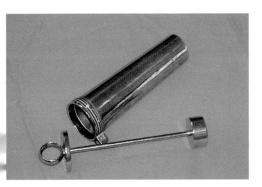

53. This instrument is commonly found in the labour suite.

a. What is this instrument?
b. For which procedure is it used?
c. What is the indication for this procedure?

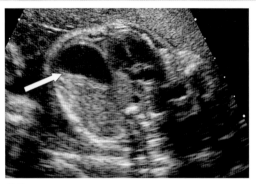

54. This ultrasound image shows a transverse section through a fetal chest.

a. Which structure is indicated by the arrow?

b. What is the diagnosis?

c. What is the overall survival rate for this condition if there are no other abnormalities in the baby?

55. This baby was found to have severe skin scarring at delivery.

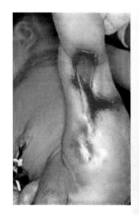

a. Which fetomaternal infection may cause this appearance?

b. Which antenatal intervention may reduce the incidence of fetal damage?

c. Name two other congenital abnormalities that may result from this fetal infection.

56. This kidney and ureter were dissected from a fetus after the pregnancy was terminated at 23 weeks' gestation. The other kidney had the same appearance.

a. How would you describe this kidney?
b. What abnormality of liquor volume might have been found on ultrasound scan?
c. What might the postmortem report have said about the fetal lungs?

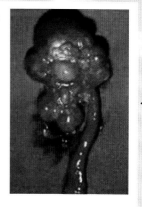

57. This is an ultrasound scan of a fetal abdomen at 15 weeks' gestation.

a. What structure is herniating through the fetal abdominal wall?
b. What is the diagnosis?
c. Which chromosomal abnormality is most commonly associated with this finding?

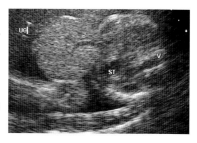

58. This newborn infant has Down syndrome.

a. Which subtle feature of Down syndrome is shown here?
b. What routine screening tests are available for this condition in pregnancy?
c. Name six features on a 20-week scan that point to the diagnosis.

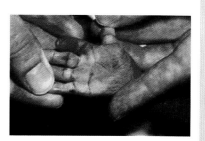

59. This baby was born weighing 2.3 kg at 39 weeks' gestation. His mother was induced for hypertension and proteinuria.

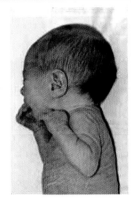

a. How would you describe this baby?
b. What is the underlying pathology?
c. Name three ultrasound features you might expect to find with this diagnosis.

60. This baby has very short and deformed long bones.

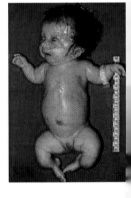

a. What is the term given to this group of congenital abnormalities?
b. Name two investigations that help make the diagnosis during pregnancy.
c. What is the main reason these babies die?

61. This baby was born to a woman who declined antenatal screening.

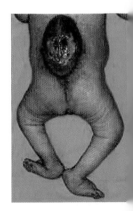

a. What abnormality is shown here?
b. Name four problems that this child might face in later life.
c. What are the two reasons for the falling incidence of this condition at birth?

62. This baby has suffered birth trauma.

a. What is this finding called?
b. What was the most likely mode of delivery?
c. What condition is the neonate more likely to develop as a consequence of this?

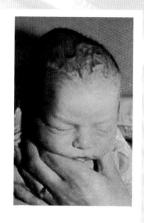

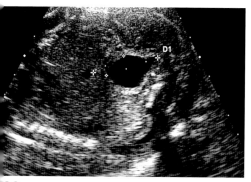

63. This ultrasound scan shows an enlarged bladder in longitudinal view. The fetus is male.

a. What is the diagnosis?
b. What are the main consequences of this condition?
c. What antenatal therapeutic intervention might be considered?

64. This is an image of a baby taken soon after delivery.

a. What physical signs are demonstrated here?
b. What do they indicate?
c. Name four possible causes for this appearance.

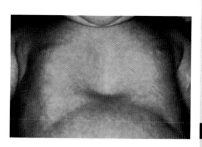

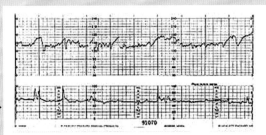

91070

65. This cardiotocogram (CTG) is taken from a low–risk woman at 40 weeks' gestation in early labour. The baseline rate was 140 beats/min.

a. How would you describe it?
b. Should monitoring be continued?
c. What alternative method of fetal monitoring can be used to monitor the fetus in labour?

66. This is a partogram taken from a multiparous woman in spontaneous labour.

a. What abnormal pattern of labour is illustrated here?
b. Name three causes for this.
c. What is the main risk if labour is allowed to continue?

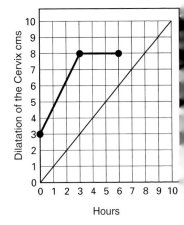

67. This pregnant woman complains of paraesthesia and numbness in the distribution shown in the picture.

a. What is the diagnosis?
b. Which nerve is involved?
c. What two treatments would you offer?

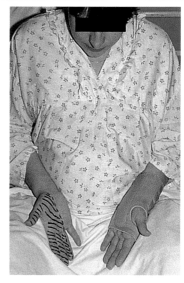

68. This woman attends a joint medical/obstetric clinic.

a. What condition does she suffer from?
b. What blood tests might you perform to confirm the diagnosis?
c. Name four complications associated with this condition in pregnancy.

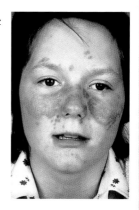

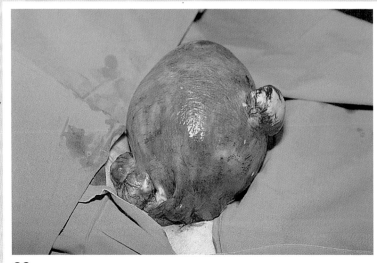

69. This was the appearance of a term uterus at caesarean section.

a. What are the structures attached to the uterus?
b. Name three complications of these in pregnancy.
c. Would you remove them at the time of the caesarean delivery?

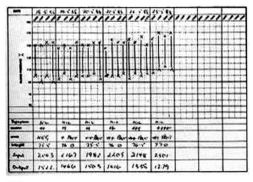

70. This is the maternal observations chart from a primiparous woman admitted at term.

a. What is the likely diagnosis?
b. Name five investigations that should be carried out.
c. What is the definitive treatment?

71. This CT scan was performed 6 weeks after delivery by caesarean section.

a. What structure has been imaged, and which view are we seeing?
b. Which obstetric measurements are shown by the dotted lines?
c. Is this test of any value in managing future pregnancies?

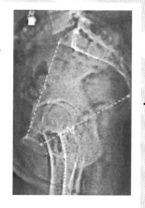

72. This woman presented at term with vulval soreness and contractions.

a. What is the diagnosis?
b. What information is critical in deciding mode of delivery?
c. What risks does a vaginal delivery pose to the baby?

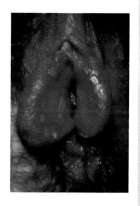

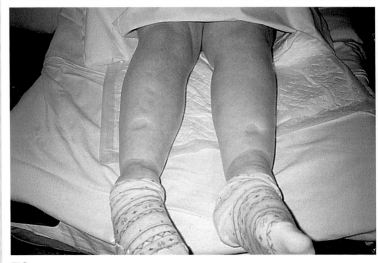

73. This woman is at 36 weeks' gestation.

a. What physical sign is evident from this image?

b. Name four other important features on examination of this patient.

c. Name five investigations that you would organize.

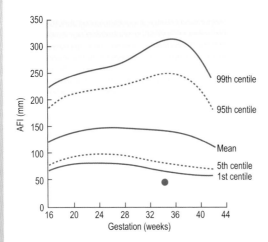

74. Study this amniotic fluid index (AFI) chart.

a. What abnormality is represented here?

b. Name three causes for this.

c. What three other features would you examine on scan?

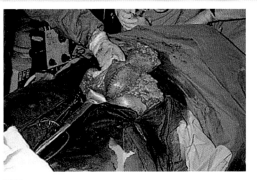

75. This image shows a uterus at the end of a caesarean section.

a. What type of caesarean section has been performed?
b. Name one immediate and one long-term complication that are more likely than after a normal caesarean section?
c. Name two valid indications for this operation.

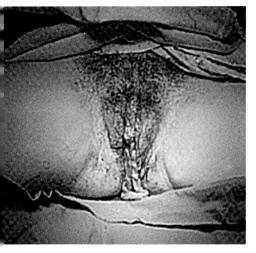

76. This woman has been rushed in from home by her midwife who attended her following spontaneous membrane rupture.

a. What problem is shown here?
b. Name four predisposing factors.
c. What are the two measures that should be taken once the patient is in hospital if the cervix is not fully dilated and the fetus is alive?

77. This young boy attended an antenatal clinic with his pregnant mother. He has a cough and very red cheeks.

a. What is the diagnosis for his infectious illness?
b. How would you ascertain if his mother is at risk of contracting the same viral illness?
c. What risks does this pose to her pregnancy?

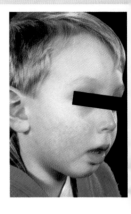

78. This image shows a transverse section through a fetal head.

a. What type of investigation has been performed?
b. Does it involve any risk to the fetus?
c. Is a CT scan a viable alternative?

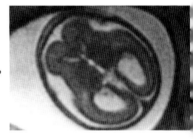

79. These cells are derived from amniotic fluid.

a. What molecular test has been performed?
b. What kind of abnormalities is it able to detect?
c. Are these cells normal? Justify your answer.

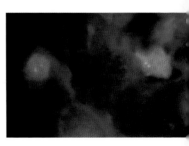

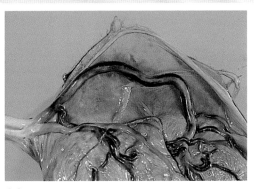

80. Following delivery this placenta was examined closely by the midwife.

a. What is this appearance called?
b. What significance may it have?
c. How might this problem present in labour?

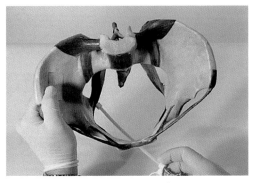

81. This image shows the bony pelvis.

a. Which structure is being pointed to?
b. Which nerve passes close to this point?
c. Why is this of importance in obstetrics?

Time	Meal and insulin dose	Capillary glucose values
0800 h		9.3 mmol/L (167.4 mg/dL)
0905 h	Breakfast and 18 units quick acting insulin	
1000 h		3.0 mmol/L (54.0 mg/dL)
1230 h		5.6 mmol/L (100.8 mg/dL)
1235 h	Lunch and 24 units quick acting insulin	
1530 h		7.2 mmol/L (129.6 mg/dL)
1800 h		4.8 mmol/L (86.4 mg/dL)
1805 h	Evening meal and 26 units quick acting insulin	
2000 h		6.9 mmol/L (124.2 mg/dL)
2200 h		5.6 mmol/L (91.8 mg/dL)
2230 h	Bedtime snack and 16 units intermediate acting insulin	
Glucose and insulin profile of a diabetic patient at 32 weeks in pregnancy		

82. Study this blood glucose profile of a diabetic patient at 32 weeks' gestation. It is representative of her profiles for the preceding week.

a. What would you do with the evening dose of long-acting insulin?
b. How would you alter her morning insulin dose?
c. How would you measure her longer-term control?

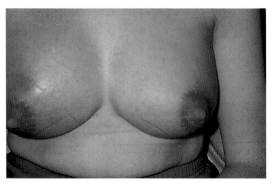

83. This woman presents with painful breastfeeding 8 days after delivery.

a. What is the diagnosis?
b. Which two species of microorganism are commonly responsible?
c. Name three components of the management.

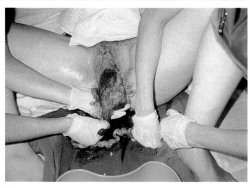

84. This image was taken during the third stage of labour.

a. What is the name of the technique which has just been used?
b. Name two complications that can occur if it is done incorrectly.
c. What is the reason this may be unsuccessful?

85. This hysterectomy was performed following a complication in labour.

a. What uterine problem is shown here?
b. Name two predisposing factors.
c. Name four ways in which it may present in labour.

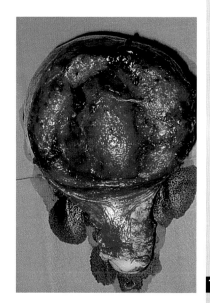

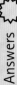

1. a. Polyhydramnios.
    b. Diabetes in pregnancy, structural abnormalities (e.g. bowel atresias, congenital diaphragmatic hernia), twin–twin transfusion syndrome, viral infections, isoimmunization.
    c. Abdominal discomfort and preterm uterine tightenings. On palpation the uterus would be large-for-dates and the fetal parts difficult to feel.

2. a. Ectopic pregnancy. The uterus is empty despite an hCG value well above the 1500 IU/L threshold at which an intrauterine gestation sac should be seen. Furthermore, there is a mass in the adnexal region.
    b. Previous ectopic pregnancy, tubal surgery, previous pelvic infection, assisted conception, intrauterine contraceptive devices.
    c. Surgical management can be open, but preferably laparoscopic. The tube can be conserved (salpingotomy) or removed entirely (salpingectomy). Small ectopics can sometimes be treated medically with methotrexate.

3. a. Gestational trophoblastic disease (molar pregnancy).
    b. A multicystic or 'snowstorm' appearance in the placenta.
    c. The patient would need to be registered with the nearest specialist trophoblast centre. Serial monitoring of serum/urine hCG measurements would be necessary. If levels failed to fall to zero, then further curettage or chemotherapy would be indicated.

4. a. Crown–rump length (CRL).
    b. The error is ±5 days using the CRL to date a pregnancy.
    c. The biparietal diameter and femur length.

5. a. The yolk sac.
    b. It is first visible at 5 weeks' gestation with a transvaginal scan and has usually gone by 12 weeks.
    c. It plays a major role in embryonic nutrition, biosynthesis and haemopoiesis.

6. a. The biparietal diameter.
    b. The choroid plexus.
    c. It produces cerebrospinal fluid.

7. a. The cerebellum.
    b. Image A shows a normal cerebellum (two hemispheres and a midline vermis).
    c. Image B shows a 'banana'-shaped cerebellum associated with neural tube defects. Other cranial ultrasound features associated with spina bifida include a 'lemon'-shaped head and an effaced cisterna magna.

8. *a.* This scan shows four amniotic sacs, suggesting a quadruplet pregnancy. Two of the membranes are thick and have lambda signs. One of the membranes is much thinner and there is no lambda sign. This suggests that there is a pair of monochorionic twins and two 'singletons'.
   b. Assisted conception (in vitro fertilization).
   c. Miscarriage, preterm labour, fetal growth restriction, pre-eclampsia, fetal anomalies, twin–twin transfusion syndrome, malpresentation and need for caesarean delivery.

9. *a.* The nuchal translucency (NT).
   b. The most common reason for NT scanning is to screen for Down syndrome.
   c. NT scanning cannot be performed after approximately 13 weeks' gestation and is still not widely available. Double or triple serum screening should be offered to all pregnant women at 15-19 weeks' gestation, although it is less sensitive as a screening test for Down syndrome than NT scanning.

10. *a.* Anencephaly (a form of neural tube defect).
   b. Serum screening at 15-19 weeks has a greater than 90% sensitivity for detection of open neural tube defects, and routine detailed scanning at 20 weeks' gestation detects more than 98% of these abnormalities.
   c. Anencephalic pregnancies are often complicated by polyhydramnios, possibly due to a failure of fetal drinking secondary to disturbed neurological function.

11. *a.* Edward syndrome.
   b. Trisomy 18.
   c. Other abnormalities commonly associated with trisomy 18 include congenital heart disease (in particular ventricular septal defect), omphalocele (found in 25%), neural tube defects, diaphragmatic hernia and rocker-bottom feet.

12. *a.* Exomphalos (omphalocele).
   b. Fetal karyotyping by either amniocentesis or chorionic villus sampling. Approximately 25% are associated with chromosomal abnormalities.
   c. Trisomies 18 and 13 are the most common aneuploidies found with exomphalos.

13. *a.* The 'double-bubble' sign.
   b. Duodenal atresia results in an enlarged fluid-filled stomach and proximal duodenum, separated by the pylorus.
   c. Down syndrome (trisomy 21) is found in 30% of cases.

14. *a.* Reduced (absent) baseline variability, late decelerations and absence of accelerations.
   b. Pathological (i.e. more than one abnormal feature).

c. Fresh meconium. This CTG is highly suggestive of fetal hypoxia and acidosis. It is very possible that this fetus has passed fresh meconium in response.

15. a. Turner syndrome (45, XO).
b. Short stature, neck webbing, cardiac abnormalities (bicuspid aortic valve, coarctation of the aorta), renal anomalies (e.g. horseshoe kidney) and streak ovaries (causing failure of secondary sexual development).
c. A cystic hygroma (collections of lymph in the posterolateral aspect of the neck).

16. a. Left facial nerve palsy.
b. Forceps delivery is most likely, although unexplained facial nerve palsies are occasionally seen after normal births.
c. No. The prognosis is very good, with the vast majority settling spontaneously within a few days.

17. a. Hypoxic ischaemic encephalopathy (HIE).
b. Electroencephalogram.
c. Babies at the moderate to severe end of the spectrum of HIE (grades II and III) have a 50–90% risk of neurodevelopmental damage.

18. a. Necrotizing enterocolitis.
b. Administration of steroids (dexamethasone or betamethasone) to the mother at least 48 h before delivery.
c. Intravenous antibiotics and fluids. Nil intake by mouth.

19. a. Occipital encephalocele.
b. Neural tube defects.
c. Ultrasound and MRI.

20. a. Fetal hydrops.
b. A, abdominal wall oedema; B, ascites.
c. Isoimmunization, chromosomal abnormalities, viral infections, fetomaternal haemorrhage, cardiac abnormalities (e.g. arrhythmias), skeletal dysplasias, twin–twin transfusion, inborn errors of metabolism, haemoglobinopathies.

21. a. Epicanthic folds, Brushfield's spots (on the iris) and upward-slanting palpebral fissures.
b. Down syndrome (trisomy 21).
c. Most cases of Down syndrome are spontaneous. The recurrence risk is quoted as 1 in 100, unless the woman's age-related risk is higher than this, in which case it is used instead. Rare forms of translocation Down syndrome may result from a parental balanced translocation. The recurrence risk is then significantly higher.

22. *a.* Umbilical artery Doppler waveform recording and measurement.
b. This waveform correlates with resistance to blood flow through the fetal side of the placenta. The presence of end-diastolic forward flow means that placental resistance is not severely elevated.
c. Pre-eclampsia occurs because of suboptimal placentation. Inadequate remodelling of maternal spiral arteries in the uterine bed leaves them as high-resistance vessels. This in turn impacts on the development of the fetal side of the placenta, also causing greater resistance to blood flow.

23. *a.* Erb's palsy.
b. Stretching or avulsion of the C5, C6 and C7 nerve roots of the brachial plexus due to excessive lateral traction at the time of delivery of the fetal shoulders.
c. Maternal diabetes mellitus (pre-existing or gestational) is a risk factor for shoulder dystocia (and therefore Erb's palsy), independent of fetal size.

24. *a.* Chickenpox (varicella zoster).
b. Maternal infection before 20 weeks' gestation carries a 1-2% risk of congenital varicella syndrome (microcephaly, seizures, neurodevelopment delay, limb hypoplasia and scarring). Infections close to delivery carry a risk of potentially very damaging neonatal chickenpox.
c. Chickenpox pneumonitis may occur with adult infections and is thought to carry a greater mortality risk in pregnancy.

25. *a.* Grade IV (major) placenta praevia (i.e. covering the internal cervical os).
b. Antepartum or intrapartum haemorrhage, abnormal lie, failure of engagement of the presenting part.
c. Previous placenta praevia, previous caesarean section, uterine anomalies, multiple gestations, high parity.

26. *a.* Potter's facies.
b. Prolonged fetal exposure to very low liquor volumes from an early gestation as a result of renal agenesis, polycystic or dysplastic kidneys or prolonged preterm ruptured membranes.
c. Pulmonary hypoplasia. Severely reduced levels of amniotic fluid prevent lung expansion and growth in utero, leading to inadequate pulmonary development.

27. *a.* Filshie clip sterilization.
b. Complications include failure (1 in 300) and regret. If it is done laparoscopically there is also a risk of visceral injury during the procedure.
c. Sterilization can be performed at the time of caesarean section and is usually carried out by removing segments of each tube and ligating the ends. The failure rate is higher (1 in 200).

28. *a.* Choroid plexus cysts.
   b. It is most closely associated with trisomy 18 (Edward syndrome). However, it also probably has a weak association with trisomy 21 (Down syndrome).
   c. 1% of normal fetuses.

29. *a.* Ventouse delivery.
   b. The site of the cup placement over the anterior aspect of the head indicates that the fetus must have been in an occipitoposterior position. It is likely that the individual performing the delivery incorrectly took the position to be occipitoanterior.
   c. Other injuries include cephalohaematomas, subgaleal haemorrhage, tentorial and venous sinus tears and subconjunctival and retinal haemorrhages. Jaundice is also more common.

30. *a.* Macrosomic.
   b. Maternal impaired glucose tolerance or diabetes mellitus.
   c. Neonatal hypoglycaemia, respiratory distress, hypocalcaemia, polycythaemia and jaundice.

31. *a.* Absent end-diastolic flow (AEDF).
   b. Increased resistance to blood flow through the placental bed secondary to placental disease.
   c. AEDF is a marker of increased perinatal morbidity and mortality. At this relatively advanced gestation it would usually indicate the need for delivery. In a compromised fetus, planned caesarean birth may be safer than an induced vaginal delivery.

32. *a.* Ophthalmia neonatorum.
   b. Chlamydia and gonorrhoea can both cause this appearance.
   c. Microbiological swabs from the eyes followed by antibiotic eye drops. Triple swabs should be taken from the woman and her partner at a genitourinary clinic and contact tracing should be carried out.

33. *a.* Bilateral talipes equinovarus ('club foot').
   b. Talipes can occur in isolation but is also associated with many chromosomal and single gene disorders, as well as multiple malformation syndromes of uncertain cause. Trisomy 18 and neuromuscular disorders are of particular note.
   c. Mild cases can be treated by physiotherapy alone. In a case of this severity, serial casting is first performed to help stretch contracted tissues prior to surgery. Ligaments are released and tendons lengthened to allow bony repositioning.

34. *a.* Congenital diaphragmatic hernia.
   b. Cardiac deviation to the right and visualization of bowel contents in the chest on the left can be seen at a 20-week routine scan in most

cases. Polyhydramnios can result if the bowel in the chest becomes obstructed. This may have presented clinically.

   c. Approximately 70%. Even in the absence of other congenital abnormalities or aneuploidy, a proportion of infants will not make it to surgery due to secondary pulmonary hypoplasia. Of those that do, the outlook is much more favourable, with the majority surviving.

35. *a.* Hydrops fetalis.
   b. Rhesus D isoimmunization.
   c. Cardiac structural abnormalities and arrhythmias, chromosomal abnormalities, fetal anaemia from other causes (e.g. haemoglobinopathies, chronic fetomaternal haemorrhage), single gene disorders, viral infections and metabolic disorders.

36. *a.* Prolonged bradycardia.
   b. Uterine hyperstimulation secondary to excessive oxytocin.
   c. Turn the woman into left lateral, turn off the oxytocin and administer a tocolytic (e.g. ritodrine intravenously or terbutaline subcutaneously). The baby will need to be delivered urgently if the bradycardia persists.

37. *a.* Gastroschisis.
   b. Exomphalos (omphalocele).
   c. A membrane surrounds most omphaloceles (unlike gastroschisis) and the bowel contents herniate into the base of the umbilical cord. The cord usually inserts into the abdominal wall to the left side of a gastroschisis.

38. *a.* Prune belly syndrome.
   b. Posterior urethral valves within the urethra of a male fetus may obstruct flow of urine, causing massive bladder dilatation. This grossly distends the abdominal wall in utero. If the bladder ruptures, or if the outflow obstruction is overcome, the abdominal wall deflates, leaving this characteristic appearance.
   c. Irreversible renal damage is likely to have occurred because of excessive retrograde pressure causing dysplastic changes.

39. *a.* Amniotic band syndrome.
   b. Anencephaly, encephalocele, facial clefts, limb amputations, fusion of digits and anterior abdominal wall defects.
   c. Very low, although cases have been reported in association with certain inherited connective tissue disorders.

40. *a.* The middle cerebral artery (MCA).
   b. Compensatory mechanisms in a growth-restricted infant cause a reduction in resistance to blood flow through the brain. The waveform in the MCA takes on a low-resistance profile until a point close to fetal death, at which point this pattern reverses.
   c. In anaemic fetuses, the maximum velocity of blood flow within the MCA increases outside of the normal range.

41. *a.* Discordant.

b. Uteroplacental insufficiency is more common in multiple gestations and may result in unequal growth patterns between the two fetuses. Alternatively, in monochorionic twin pregnancies, twin–twin transfusion syndrome may produce a larger 'recipient' twin and smaller 'donor' twin.

c. A growth-restricted newborn is at greater risk of perinatal asphyxia, meconium aspiration syndrome, necrotizing enterocolitis, hypothermia, hypoglycaemia and jaundice.

42. *a.* Lumbosacral meningocele (spina bifida).

b. Other common ultrasound features include 'lemon'-shaped skull, Arnold–Chiari malformation ('banana' cerebellum and effacement of cisterna magna) and talipes.

c. Neural tube defects demonstrate polygenic inheritance. The recurrence risk after one affected pregnancy is 2-3%. This can be reduced to less than 1% by taking periconceptual high-dose folic acid (5 mg daily).

43. *a.* Pathological. The baseline variability is <5 beats/min, and there are no accelerations (unreactive). There are no decelerations and the baseline rate is normal.

b. Emergency caesarean section.

c. It would be very likely with this history and this CTG to find a severe metabolic acidosis in both the umbilical artery and vein.

44. *a.* The horns of the lateral ventricles.

b. Ventriculomegaly. Hydrocephalus is a term reserved for this finding in association with increased head circumference.

c. Chromosomal abnormalities, neural tube defects, congenital infections (cytomegalovirus and toxoplasmosis), congenital stenosis of the aqueduct and a host of less common malformation syndromes. A normal outcome is possible, especially with very borderline cases.

45. *a.* Intraventricular haemorrhage (blood is seen as the white areas in the lateral ventricles).

b. The preterm and growth-restricted infant is at greater risk of this complication, in particular if superadded perinatal hypoxia or acidosis occurs.

c. Depending on the severity of the intraventricular haemorrhage, the consequences range from none to hydrocephalus and permanent neurodevelopmental damage.

46. *a.* Forceps delivery.

b. Suspected or confirmed fetal compromise (CTG abnormalities/fresh meconium/low scalp pH value) or maternal medical reasons contraindicating the Valsalva manoeuvre (pushing) (e.g. berry aneurysms, recent intracranial bleeds, cardiac abnormalities, retinal detachments).

c. Facial bruising, facial nerve palsy, skull fracture, maternal soft tissue damage.

47. a. 45, XO.
  b. Turner syndrome.
  c. Short stature, coarctation of the aorta, streak ovaries, infertility, renal anomalies.

48. a. Multicystic.
  b. The visualization of the bladder and normal levels of amniotic fluid.
  c. Multicystic dysplastic kidney (MCDK). Most inherited cystic renal conditions involve both kidneys (e.g. infantile and adult polycystic kidney disease). Early obstruction is one possible cause for MCDK. Bilateral MCDK carries a poor prognosis.

49. a. Silastic ventouse cup.
  b. No. The design of this ventouse cup does not allow for its placement over the flexion point when the fetus is in an occipitoposterior position. Specially constructed 'OP' cups are required for a rotational ventouse delivery.
  c. Medical conditions that predispose to fetal bleeding problems are strict contraindications. Haemophilia or fetal thrombocytopenia (e.g. secondary to alloimmue thrombocytopenia or maternal idiopathic thrombocytopenia) are examples.

50. a. Cystic hygroma.
  b. Turner syndrome (45, XO) is the most common cause. Noonan, Robert's and multiple pterygium syndromes are other much less common causes.
  c. Karyotyping (amniocentesis or chorionic villus sampling).

51. a. Herpes simplex and varicella zoster.
  b. Hepatosplenomegaly, thrombocytopenia, meningoencephalitis, pneumonitis and disseminated intravascular coagulation. Long-term neurodevelopmental damage is common amongst survivors.
  c. Aciclovir.

52. a. Necrotizing enterocolitis.
  b. Respiratory distress syndrome, intraventricular haemorrhage, periventricular leukomalacia, chronic lung disease, retinopathy of prematurity.
  c. Administration of antenatal steroids (betamethasone or dexamethasone) at least 48 h before delivery.

53. a. Amnioscope.
  b. Fetal blood sampling during labour.
  c. This procedure is indicated when a CTG becomes pathological in labour (i.e. it has two or more abnormal features). The CTG carries a high false-positive rate for fetal acidosis and hypoxia. Relying solely on the

IN *focus* **Answers**

CTG during labour as an indicator of fetal well-being would result in excessive numbers of unnecessary caesarean sections for presumed fetal compromise.

54. *a.* Fetal stomach.
  b. Congenital diaphragmatic hernia.
  c. Pulmonary hypoplasia is the main limiting factor for survival in this condition if there are no other anomalies. If the neonate can be oxygenated satisfactorily then the outlook is quite good, with approximately 70% survival rates. Failure to achieve adequate ventilation is associated with an extremely poor prognosis.

55. *a.* Varicella zoster (chickenpox).
  b. Giving intravenous immunoglobulin to exposed non-immune pregnant women reduces maternal and fetal infection rates.
  c. Other anomalies found with the congenital varicella syndrome include microcephaly, limb hypoplasia and eye defects.

56. *a.* Multicystic.
  b. Oligo- or anhydramnios.
  c. If renal function was reduced enough to result in very low or absent liquor volumes, then the inability of the fetal lungs to expand in utero is likely to have caused pulmonary hypoplasia.

57. *a.* Liver.
  b. Exomphalos (omphalocele).
  c. Trisomy 18 most commonly, but also trisomy 13.

58. *a.* Single palmar crease.
  b. Nuchal translucency scanning at 11-13 weeks. The addition of first trimester biochemistry to the nuchal scan results in the 'combined' test. Serum biochemistry at 15-19 weeks is known as the 'double', 'triple' or 'quadruple' test, depending on how many markers are measured. Measuring all these variables is called the 'integrated' test.
  c. Cardiac defects (especially atrioventricular septal defect), duodenal atresia, echogenic bowel, ≥6 mm nuchal fold, clinodactyly, short femur, sandal gap and possibly renal pelvic dilatation and choroid plexus cysts.

59. *a.* Growth-restricted.
  b. Uteroplacental insufficiency secondary to pre-eclampsia.
  c. Asymmetry between abdominal circumference (AC) and head circumference measurements. Slowing of the progression of AC values over serial scans. Oligohydramnios and raised resistance patterns in the umbilical artery Doppler waveforms.

60. *a.* Skeletal dysplasias.
  b. Ultrasound and molecular genetics.
  c. Pulmonary hypoplasia and respiratory distress due to a small chest.

61. *a.* Lumbosacral myelomeningocele (spina bifida).
   b. Motor problems (may be wheelchair-bound), bladder and bowel incontinence and hydrocephalus (which may need to be surgically shunted and may result in neurodevelopmental delay).
   c. The increased use of folic acid around the time of conception has reduced the actual incidence of these conditions. Almost universal detection through maternal serum α-fetoprotein testing and routine detailed scanning at 20 weeks means that most couples with an affected pregnancy have a choice regarding termination.

62. *a.* Cephalohaematoma.
   b. This is more likely with a ventouse delivery.
   c. Jaundice is more likely because of the increased bilirubin resulting from haemolysis of the red cells within the haematoma.

63. *a.* Posterior urethral valves (dilated thick walled bladder with 'keyhole' posterior urethral expansion).
   b. Increased pressure in the renal tract usually causes some degree of pelvicalyceal dilatation and commonly results in dysplastic changes in the renal parenchyma and reduced function. A marked reduction in amniotic fluid is probable, followed by secondary pulmonary hypoplasia.
   c. If liquor volumes decline before 32 weeks' gestation and fetal renal function is preserved, then pigtail catheters may be sited through the bladder in utero to bypass the obstruction.

64. *a.* Subcostal and sternal recession.
   b. Respiratory distress/compromise.
   c. Hyaline membrane disease (associated with prematurity), transient tachypnoea of the newborn, congenital pneumonia, pneumothorax, pulmonary hypoplasia.

65. *a.* Reactive (normal). There are accelerations on a normal baseline with good variability. There are no decelerations.
   b. No. Low-risk women do not need to be continuously monitored by CTG in labour.
   c. Fetal monitoring should be continued in all labours, namely by intermittent auscultation every 15 min with a Pinard stethoscope or hand-held Doppler. In second stage, the fetal heart should be auscultated after every contraction. The colour of the liquor draining is another (insensitive) method of intrapartum fetal surveillance.

66. *a.* Secondary arrest.
   b. Dysfunctional uterine activity, true cephalopelvic disproportion, malposition (e.g. occipitoposterior) or malpresentation (e.g. face, shoulder or brow).
   c. If an obstruction is not overcome, then secondary arrest may finally result in uterine rupture in a multiparous patient. Great care must therefore be taken in using oxytocin in this situation.

67. *a.* Carpal tunnel syndrome.
 b. Median nerve.
 c. Splinting and simple analgesics if there is pain. There is no role for diuretics in pregnancy, and the need for surgery is very rare.

68. *a.* Systemic lupus erythematosus.
 b. Baseline full blood count and renal biochemistry should be performed. An autoantibody profile should also be requested.
 c. The effect of lupus on pregnancy depends on the extent of visceral organ involvement, levels of disease activity and which autoantibodies are present. Anti-Ro and anti-La antibodies, if found, may cause fetal heart block. Anticardioplin antibodies and lupus anticoagulant are associated with an increased risk of miscarriage, abruption, fetal growth restriction, pre-eclampsia and maternal thrombosis, as are renal involvement and hypertension.

69. *a.* Serosal fibroids.
 b. Fibroids often enlarge in pregnancy. If they outgrow their blood supply, then a process called red degeneration may occur. This can cause significant pain, as can torsion of a pedunculated fibroid. Submucous fibroids may obstruct the lower part of the uterus and cause malpresentation. Fibroids predispose to primary postpartum haemorrhage.
 c. No. Myomectomy at the time of caesarean section is hazardous and best avoided. Bleeding can be torrential and difficult to control.

70. *a.* Pre-eclampsia (proteinuric hypertension of pregnancy).
 b. Renal function tests, 24-h urine collection for total protein estimation, liver function tests, fetal ultrasound and platelet count.
 c. Delivery of the fetus and placenta.

71. *a.* A lateral view of the female pelvis (pelvimetry).
 b. The upper dotted line is called the 'true conjugate' and measures the anteroposterior diameter at the inlet. The lower dotted line measures the same, at the outlet.
 c. No. Pelvimetry was previously performed during pregnancy to help predict the chances of successful breech vaginal delivery. Women having an emergency caesarean section often underwent pelvimetry to help advise about future deliveries. Good-quality evidence shows that pelvimetry is not a helpful investigation in either of these scenarios.

72. *a.* Vulval herpes.
 b. Is this the first ever attack (primary herpes) or a recurrence?
 c. If this represents a recurrence, then the risk of neonatal herpes following a vaginal delivery is very low because of passive immunity from maternal antibodies. Primary herpes occurring any time after 30 weeks is an indication for caesarean section because transmission rates to the fetus born vaginally are much higher.

73. a. Pitting peripheral oedema.

b. Blood pressure, reflexes, presence of clonus, upper abdominal tenderness and uterine size.

c. If there is concern regarding the possibility of pre-eclampsia, maternal investigations should include 24-h urine collection for protein, midstream urine culture, liver and renal biochemistry (including urate), full blood count and occasionally clotting profile. Fetal investigations include CTG, growth parameters, liquor volume and umbilical artery Doppler waveform measurements.

74. a. Oligohydramnios.

b. Uteroplacental insufficiency (e.g. pre-eclampsia), rupture of membranes and severe bilateral fetal renal abnormalities.

c. Fetal growth parameters and umbilical artery Doppler should help to identify a placental pathology. Abnormally dilated or multicystic kidneys will point to a renal cause. The diagnosis of ruptured membranes must be made clinically.

75. a. Classical caesarean section (vertical incision).

b. Blood loss is greater with classical caesarean section and the risk of uterine rupture is higher in a subsequent pregnancy.

c. Inadequate access to the lower segment (e.g. fibroids, severe adhesions and placenta percreta) and malpresentations with reduced liquor at preterm gestations.

76. a. Cord prolapse.

b. Prematurity, malpresentations, polyhydramnios, multiple gestations and artificial rupture of membranes with a 'high head'.

c. The cord should be gently held in a cupped hand in the vagina with the fingers pressing on the presenting part to relieve any pressure on it. The woman should adopt the 'knees-to-chest' position until emergency caesarean section can be performed.

77. a. Slapped cheek syndrome (erythema infectiosum). Caused by parvovirus B12.

b. Many adult parvovirus B12 infections are asymptomatic. Serological testing for IgM antibodies raised against parvovirus would recognize a recent maternal infection. IgG antibodies usually indicate past maternal infection.

c. Fetal infection with parvovirus B12 can cause an aplastic crisis, resulting in fetal anaemia, hydrops and intrauterine fetal death.

78. a. Fetal MRI.

b. There is no evidence that MRI harms pregnancies.

c. No. CT scanning involves very high fetal exposures to ionizing radiation which early on in pregnancy may increase the risk of congenital abnormalities and later may have an impact on growth, neurological development and future risk of malignancy.

79. a. Fluorescent in situ hybridization (FISH) following amniocentesis.
b. Abnormalities of chromosome number (e.g. trisomies).
c. This cell is normal because there are two signals per cell. Only if this were a Y chromosome probe would it be an abnormal cell.

80. a. Vasa praevia.
b. The vessels running through the membranes form part of the fetal circulation. If they tear, fetal exsanguination can occur very quickly.
c. The time of highest risk for fetal bleeding due to vasa praevia occurs when the membranes rupture spontaneously or if artificial rupture is performed. Vaginal bleeding occurs and the fetal heart tracing becomes abnormal in the absence of maternal shock.

81. a. The ischial spine.
b. The pudendal nerve.
c. A pudendal nerve block can be easily carried out by an obstetrician in second stage to provide fast-acting and safe analgesia sufficient for a forceps delivery or repair of an extensive vaginal and perineal tear.

82. a. Increase it. The fasting glucose level in the morning is too high and usually reflects inadequate insulin overnight.
b. Decrease it. The post breakfast blood glucose is a little low. Warnings of hypoglycaemia are less pronounced in pregnancy and even a long-standing experienced diabetic may nevertheless be caught out by this.
c. By measuring glycosylated haemoglobin (HbA_{1c}). A value less than 7% suggests reasonable recent sugar control.

83. a. Mastitis.
b. *Staphylococcus* and *Streptococcus* species.
c. The woman should be encouraged to express milk from that side and to continue breastfeeding with the other. Flucloxacillin is the empiric treatment of choice. Nipple swabs or expressed milk can be sent for microbiological culture and sensitivity testing. Non-steroidal anti-inflammatory drugs can be used for analgesia. Expert help with breastfeeding technique should reduce the chances of sore nipples and recurrences of the same problem.

84. a. Controlled cord traction.
b. Uterine inversion can occur if excessive cord traction is used, particularly if the uterus is somewhat atonic. This obstetric complication causes profound bradycardic shock, which is corrected by replacing the uterine fundus as soon as possible. Placental cotyledons may be retained if this technique is poorly performed.
c. 1-2% of placentas remain adherent to the uterine wall despite controlled cord traction. They are removed manually in theatre under regional or general anaesthesia. Much less commonly the placenta is morbidly adherent and cannot be removed, even manually. A hysterectomy is usually necessary.

85.
  a. Uterine rupture.

  b. Previous caesarean section (especially classical) and any other full-thickness uterine damage (e.g. myomectomy or perforation at the time of curettage). Obstructed labour in multiparous women and the injudicious use of oxytocin are other causes.

  c. It may present as severe continuous suprapubic pain, maternal collapse, intrapartum vaginal bleeding, haematuria or profound and sudden CTG abnormalities.

Index